AF324334

AGE AND IDENTITY IN EIGHTEENTH-CENTURY ENGLAND

The Body, Gender and Culture

Series Editor: *Lynn Botelho*

Titles in this Series

1 Courtly Indian Women in Late Imperial India
Angma Dey Jhala

2 Paracelsus's Theory of Embodiment: Conception and Gestation in Early Modern Europe
Amy Eisen Cislo

3 The Prostitute's Body: Rewriting Prostitution in Victorian Britain
Nina Attwood

4 Old Age and Disease in Early Modern Medicine
Daniel Schäfer

5 The Life of Madame Necker: Sin, Redemption and the Parisian Salon
Sonja Boon

6 Stays and Body Image in London: The Staymaking Trade, 1680–1810
Lynn Sorge-English

7 Prostitution and Eighteenth-Century Culture: Sex, Commerce and Morality
Ann Lewis and Markman Ellis (eds)

8 The Aboriginal Male in the Enlightenment World
Shino Konishi

9 Anatomy and the Organization of Knowledge, 1500–1850
Matthew Landers and Brian Muñoz (eds)

10 Blake, Gender and Culture
Helen P. Bruder and Tristanne J. Connolly (eds)

AGE AND IDENTITY IN EIGHTEENTH-CENTURY ENGLAND

BY

Helen Yallop

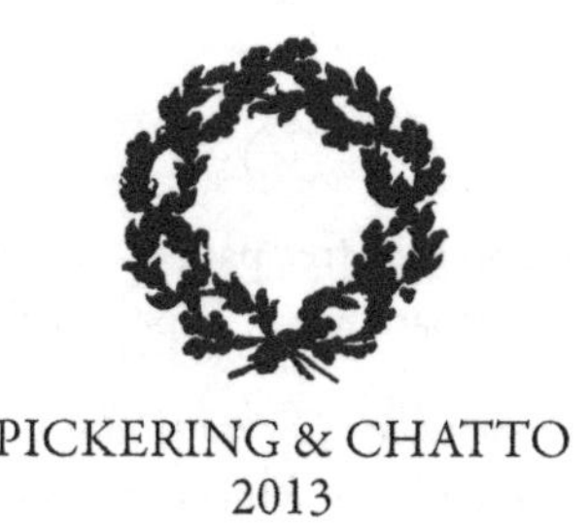

PICKERING & CHATTO

2013

Published by Pickering & Chatto (Publishers) Limited
21 Bloomsbury Way, London WC1A 2TH

2252 Ridge Road, Brookfield, Vermont 05036-9704, USA

www.pickeringchatto.com

To the best of the Publisher's knowledge every effort has been made to contact
relevant copyright holders and to clear any relevant copyright issues.
Any omissions that come to their attention will be remedied in future editions.

BRITISH LIBRARY CATALOGUING IN PUBLICATION DATA

Yallop, Helen.
Age and identity in eighteenth-century England. – (The body, gender and
culture)
1. Aging – England – History – 18th century. 2. Aging – Social aspects –
England –History – 18th century. 3. Older people – England – History – 18th
century. 4. Identity (Psychology) in old age – England – History – 18th century.
I. Title II. Series
305.2'6'0942'09033-dc23

ISBN-13: 9781848934016
e: 9781781440339

This publication is printed on acid-free paper that conforms to the American
National Standard for the Permanence of Paper for Printed Library Materials.

Typeset by Pickering & Chatto (Publishers) Limited
Printed and bound in the United Kingdom by the MPG Books Group

CONTENTS

ACKNOWLEDGEMENTS

My thanks go to Laura Gowing, Lynn Botelho, Colin Jones, Naomi Tadmor, Toni Weller, Tim Reinke-Williams, Eleanor Hooker, Matthew McCormack, Daire Carr, Ruth Ireland, Henry Yallop, Stephina Clarke, Richard Yallop, Gwyneth Yallop and my anonymous reviewers.

INTRODUCTION

In November 2010, I was asked to speak at a conference organized by the Royal Society of Medicine entitled 'Our Changing Expectations of Life: What do we Really Want?' The aims of the conference were to question why we wish for longer, healthier lives and what exactly 'aging' means in our current culture. Most of the speakers came from a scientific background, but along with a few scholars and commentators from the media and humanities, I was able to give something of an alternative perspective. Still, I was the only one at the conference who was looking to the past in order to better understand our notions of aging in the present. Despite any preconceptions I may have had about this, the response I received was overwhelmingly receptive and positive. Listeners were keen to concede that the past can give us a keen sense of what is timeless about human endeavours to control and ameliorate the aging process. Moreover – and this is the surprising part – some of my findings about eighteenth-century ideas actually reflect what is *current* in aging research. Indeed it is often the case that those from a non-academic (or simply non-historical) background who read or listen to my work are keen to tell me how surprisingly 'modern' some of the eighteenth-century views on aging appear to them, and how 'relevant' they appear today.

Readers will probably find that some of the views from the past that this book shares will sometimes feel uncannily close to what we read about aging in our society. Now, as in the eighteenth century, we live in a society where aging is vigorously researched, discussed and represented in politics, science and the media. Anti-aging is big business, whether in medical research, medical aesthetics, cosmetics, dietetics or any of the various lifestyle strategies that we may choose to pursue. Whereas the specifics of each of these is of course unique to twenty-first-century global society, there is nothing new about our fascination with aging, nor about the apparently very deep human need to try to stop it, delay, or even reverse it. As David Boyd-Haycock has shown in his *Mortal Coil: A Short History of Living Longer* (2008), the desire to extend healthy, human life has been with us since the Ancients.

In this context, perhaps the most striking idea that comes out of this study – and certainly the idea that feels most relevant to our current thinking about the management of aging – is the degree to which eighteenth-century people imagined that aging could be a matter of personal choice. Eighteenth-century writers thought that managing aging was largely a matter of what we might now refer to as positive mental attitude: they united in their faith in mind-over-matter and in their insistence that aging could be controlled through right thinking and sociable interaction. The sensational title of Tom Kirkwood's 1999 bestseller, *Time of Our Lives: Why Ageing is Neither Inevitable Nor Necessary* might suggest that there is something progressive, even futuristic, about the idea of choosing how our bodies age. But, as this book demonstrates, it is not only the current medical establishment that has taught us that aging can be a matter of choice rather than destiny.

Yet having noted how some of the ideas about aging in this book may feel 'relevant' or 'modern', it is now attendant upon me to point out that however accessible these views might be, there is nothing ahistorical about the idea of aging. Let me explain. As a universal aspect of humanity, aging seems to be something very 'natural', almost ahistorical: all people at all times have experienced aging. Yet just as historians have come to realize that past societies could have very different concepts of apparently very natural and universal things – concepts of 'the body' and of 'the self', for example – this study starts from the premise that there is nothing constant about 'aging'. Although aging is a 'natural' fundamental fact about human experience, different societies understand it in different ways and past societies have understood it and written about it in ways that are uniquely their own. The more we understand this, the more we can look critically and deeply about our own understandings and assumptions on the subject. This book looks at how one past society – England in the eighteenth century – understood aging, and explains how eighteenth-century people made sense of their aging processes.

Eighteenth-century ideas about aging were not simply different to our own, but – as I am keen to emphasize – complex, distinctive, subtle and difficult to understand without anachronism. The first point I make in Chapter 1 should go some way to preparing us for this conceptual stretch. There was no word 'aging' in the eighteenth century, no specific word dedicated to describe the process of getting older. Although it is therefore technically impossible to write about eighteenth-century concepts of 'aging', this study reconstructs a set of ideas about age, bodies, change and lifetime that was distinctive to England at this particular time.

I have chosen to call this book 'Age and Identity' because I consider 'aging' not only as a body issue, or a medical issue, but also as an aspect of personal identity. Like race, gender and class, age is a facet of personhood that gives meaning to our notions of who we are. Questions about the nature of aging are intrinsically connected to questions about the nature of personal identity, for 'aging' – being a person with a body for the course of a lifetime – is a condition of personhood. As historians we are now quite familiar with how bodies shape identities, but are arguably less attuned to how time also plays a role. As Raymond Martin and John Barresi explain, a primary condition for the philosophical problematization of personhood is an acknowledgement that it exists 'over time'.[1] Or as the father of modern personal identity theory, John Locke, explained in 1691, investigating the nature of the 'person' was essentially asking the question of 'whether a Man ... be the same Man or No, when his Body is changed'.[2] Problematizing aging is essentially a question of problematizing identity.

Working at an epistemological level, this study attempts to access the raw concept of 'aging' in the eighteenth-century mindset and its significance in an eighteenth-century world view. A broadly cultural approach is married with a history of ideas and a history of the body. Respecting the major paradigmatic shifts in the history of science and philosophy, I provide a close reading of contemporary medical and physiological texts to reveal how physicians incorporated aging within their visions of bodily function. However, the study also looks beyond the exalted realms of physiology to consider how aging was represented to the health-conscious readers of eighteenth-century England: via a burst of newly accessible and affordable print. Principally considering medical advice literature, but also periodicals, newspapers, conduct works, dictionaries and encyclopaedia, the book examines the representation of aging at a cultural moment fascinated by embodied personhood, and describes how the aging body became a lens for investigating the nature of mankind and its relationship with society.

As any Enlightenment scholar will know, the eighteenth century witnessed the proliferation of new physiological and psycho-perceptual schemes that offered profound revisions for understanding the body and the self. The most notable of these were the Cartesian-inspired body model of 'hydraulic mechanism' developed by Herman Boerhaave and the 'revolution' in personal identity theory begun by John Locke. Yet as well as these recognizably 'new' influences on understandings of age and aging there remained a host of older ones. Paradigmatic shifts in philosophical and physiological modes of thought did not automatically displace what may be understood as the more 'fundamental' ideas from cosmology and the Western Christian tradition. As such, this book respects that in many ways the eighteenth century must be seen as a period witnessing many modernizing influences, but suggests that ideas about aging were sufficiently flexible to allow the coexistence of the old and new.

In the remainder of this introductory chapter I have several goals. Firstly, I want to problematize the concept of 'aging' itself, and to underline its historical specificity. I situate my work within the existing academic approach to the history of 'aging' in socio-cultural history and the excellent work that has been done in recent years. Also, I outline very briefly the theories informing modern body studies, and those that have been influential in informing the body-centric work on England in the eighteenth-century. I then provide the cultural context for my study, describing the sources themselves and the cultural regime that enabled and endorsed them. Finally, I provide a chapter breakdown, and explain how the structure of the work contributes to its analytic value.

Age and Aging as Tools of (Historical) Analysis

'Aging', according to the current *Oxford English Dictionary*, is 'the process of growing old'. Central to our concept is the knowledge that aging is an intrinsic, developmental human process: an inevitable one-way journey. Aging is something that we can talk and write about with the conviction that it is a real phenomenon. It is part of the way that we conceive of ourselves as humans and part of the way that we make sense of the world and our experience in it.

The way that we think and talk about age and aging today is heavily influenced by the academic discipline of gerontology. Gerontology is a twentieth-century science, and its very existence is the product of being able to understand aging in peculiarly modern ways. Gerontology is the study of the social, psychological and biological aspects of aging (it is to be distinguished from geriatrics, which is the branch of medicine that studies the diseases of the elderly). Gerontologists have familiarized us with the notion that aging is a complex phenomenon, and involves the interplay of many different factors. Indeed, the definition of 'aging' in modern social gerontology is suitably and suggestively complex. It is, according to current scholarship in the field, 'the interplay of physical, psychological, and social phenomena that over time cause changes in a person's functional capacities and influence social definitions'.[3] As this rather long-winded definition might suggest, modern social gerontologists and sociologists are keen to point out that although aging may be a biological process, its greatest significance is undeniably a social one.[4] 'It is becoming harder to call age or aging purely natural', writes Margaret Morganroth Gullette, prominent among the self-styled 'age critics' of social theory.[5]

As the sociologists Sara Arber and Jay Ginn are keen to stress, recognizing the differences between the social and the biological aspects of age and aging is absolutely central to any serious academic enquiry, historical or otherwise. 'In the same way that the distinction between sex and gender became a basic tenet of feminist research in the 1970s', they write, an 'adequate' sociological theory of age needs to distinguish between at least three different meanings. Firstly, chronological (or calendar) age: this is essentially biological age measured in years or the number of years that we have lived. Closely related is 'physiological age', which is a medical construct, referring to the physical aging of the body, manifest in levels of functional impairments. For example, a person who has undergone severe stress or illness resulting in chronic damage to the body might have a chronological age of fifty years, but a 'physiological' age of sixty years.

Finally, 'social' or 'cultural' age refers to the social attitudes and behaviours seen as appropriate for a particular chronological age. Society deems what is appropriate for different stages in life. In all three meanings, Ginn and Arber are keen to underline, aging is gendered (that is, operates differently for men and women), and is also socially structured.[6]

Even if some of the nuances of such pronouncements remain pertinent at the theoretical level alone, the basic division between the broadly biological and the broadly cultural aspects of aging is one that has been influential in all scholarship on aging, including historical work. An individual's 'chronological' age is, quite simply, the number of years he or she has lived. Cultural age, by contrast, is the understanding of age according to a particular community's value system. Aging may be measured via those symbolic systems or mental maps that structure ideas about life course and the nature of time itself. As historians, we are of course aware that each society has its own cultural schedule for an individual's appropriate social progress through life, and such systems inevitably form people's fundamental assumptions about who they are.

Whereas aging, basically defined, is the process of becoming old, it does not imply that a person *is* old. As contemporary gerontologists are always keen to remind us, aging is a lifelong process.[7] A study of aging should emphasize not only the product of the aging process but also the process itself, and a history of aging should not necessarily be confined to an examination of the elderly. To some extent, 'aging' is semantically problematic, because in modern parlance it has become synonymous with oldness and old age: 'aging' – the adjective, is a judgement in itself. When discussing the parameters of this project with others (scholars or not) they tend to assume I conduct research about old people in the past. However, this work is not about old age, but about the process itself and how it was explained in eighteenth-century terms. The desire to reflect this (and indeed to avoid the troublesome variant spelling of 'ag(e)ing'), is another reason why this book claims to investigate 'age and identity'.

As such, this approach presents a considerable departure from how historians have tackled the topic of 'aging' to date. The semantic difficulty 'aging' presents has been reflected in the historiography, for the focus of historical work up till now has been on the end of life: that last isolatable period of decline, and the most obvious manifestation of getting older. In fact, within historical scholarship, 'aging' has become rather synonymous with 'old age'. In addition, the approach hitherto has been heavily socio-cultural rather than body-centric. Broadly speaking, historians have focused on the cultural significance of the older person, their representation, their experience, how they were defined, and what it meant to be 'old' in the past.

Like much early-modern socio-cultural history, interest in the history of aging began in the 1970s. In 1976, Keith Thomas delivered a paper entitled 'Age and Authority in Early Modern England'. His first sentence, 'there is nothing constant about the social meaning of age', opened the floor to the problematization of aging as a subject for historical enquiry.[8] Yet until the deconstructive turn in the 1980s, the history of the household and the family set the tone for much of the early scholarship, leading to a prioritization of issues like employment, property ownership and household authority.[9] As the title of Thomas's paper suggests, his concern was with the balance of power relations in early modern society, and the rights and obligations of different age groups. Also, overtly modern concerns about twentieth-century aging demographics surfaced quite obliquely and unapologetically in early work on the history of aging. Peter Laslett included 'A History of Aging and the Aged' in his 1977 collection of *Essays in Historical Sociology*, in which his primary focus was – in his own words – on the elderly as 'a problem to be solved'.[10] Similarly, his 1984 article, 'The Significance of the Past in the Study of Ageing', focused on the role of the elderly in kinship networks and changing demographics.[11] Laslett's *A Fresh Map of Life: The Emergence of the Third Age* (1989), was likewise written from a then-and-now perspective, and discussed the definition and institutionalization of old age as a life stage.[12] This particular trope continues to shape historical scholarship on aging, as the title of Pat Thane's *Old Age in English History: Past Experiences, Present Issues* (2000) might suggest. Therein, she states that one of the purposes of her book is to 'ask whether what is happening is so new or such a burden'.[13]

A related issue that characterized early work and continues to shape historical research into aging is the stigmatization of the elderly. Thane's work has definitely challenged assumptions about past attitudes towards old age, drawing attention, as it does, to the lack of homogeneity in early modern views. Certainly attitudes towards the elderly in early modern society were not universally negative.[14] However, as Susannah Ottaway pointed out in her recent study, a still very perceptible and pervasive desire amongst historians to understand the current stigmatization of aging has occasioned 'sweeping narratives' or 'collections of essays that bring together the history of old age in very disparate times and places'.[15]

Historians of aging often ask the question 'who was old?' and how they were accounted old in past societies. Typically, scholars have considered when and how an individual was deemed eligible to receive Poor Relief, or retire from full active economic life, implying that these factors are the determinants of 'old age' in society. More recently, attention has focused on the relative balance of 'chronological' and 'cultural' determinants in the definition of old age. Several historical studies have examined how early modern people might have defined the onset of old age, and the historical question typically posed in these contexts is whether these definitive factors might be understood as chronological or cultural. That is, was old age understood to begin at a certain point in time, or were the factors that determined someone 'old' actually dependent upon the visible trappings of old age: physical disability, wrinkles or grey hair? Ottaway has recently concurred with Thane in demonstrating that chronological age did play a significant and increasing role in determining who was 'old' in the eighteenth century; but she remains ultimately faithful to the historiographical consensus that cultural determinants remained 'at the core of the understanding of the aging process' in this period.[16] Demonstrating that oldness could be a matter of subjective, cultural judgements in past societies seems to have been a central pre-occupation for historians of old age, and these findings are typically presented as the triumph of cultural standards over biological. Lynn Botelho is often quoted for neatly stating that in the early modern period, 'a woman became old when she looked old'.[17]

More recently scholars have looked at the cultural significance, experience and representation of old age in early modern England. Prominent amongst this group are Botelho and Thane, who were first to draw explicit attention to the historical specificity of the cultural value of age and aging. In 2001 they opened their volume on *Women and Aging in British Society since 1500* stating that historians of old age were only just 'coming to grips' with 'the fact that old age is a highly nuanced process, one that is culturally embedded and not merely biological'.[18] Within the ensuing research, particular attention focused on the representation or experience of being both old and female. The work of Katherine Kitteridge on the sexualized older woman, and Botelho's own research on representations and perceptions of post-menopausal women in early modern England are prime examples.[19] Anne Kugler has done particular justice to this mode of enquiry with her phenomenal devotion to investigating the autobiographical experience of old age in the diary of Lady Sara Cowper (1644–1720).[20]

As an extension of her research into the investigation into the representation of old age, Botelho has also considered the presentation of old age as a medical condition. As she notes, historians of medicine traditionally look to paradigm shifts in physiology to explain changes in medical attitudes towards old age, and consequently to the publication of recognizably 'geriatric' or 'gerontological' texts to demonstrate its 'medicalization'. An accepted historiography of geriatric medicine locates the shift between 1850 and 1950, yet Botelho argues that the medicalization of old age began much earlier – in the late seventeenth century. It was then, she explains, that 'the elderly no longer "aged", but "suffered" from ageing and that suffering was to be mitigated by the medical practitioner'.[21]

Filling a 'yawning gap' in the historiography of aging, and focusing particularly on old age in eighteenth-century England is Ottaway's recent study, *The Decline of Life: Old Age in Eighteenth-Century England* (2004).[22] The backdrop for her study is the economic and demographic transformation associated with the onset of the Industrial Revolution. She considers the effect of these upheavals on both the lives of, and the perception of, the aged. As mortality and age at marriage dropped and fertility rose, the population of England grew both larger and younger. During the late eighteenth and early nineteenth centuries each successive generation was larger than its predecessor, the ratio of the age group '15–29' to the age group '30 and over' reaching almost 65 per cent in the late eighteenth century.[23] Coupled with a general rise in population from mid-century onwards, this preponderance of youth inevitably caused intergenerational tensions and changes in traditional age relations, which were further complicated by such social factors as decline in traditional patriarchal living arrangements.

The later eighteenth century witnessed a rise in manufacturing and growth of factory-based production that set the stage for rapid industrialization.[24] The quality of Poor Relief also declined significantly. The increasing connection between old age and poverty which Ottaway has charted throughout the century must, she argues, 'have had ramifications for general attitudes towards aging'. These attitudes, she writes, 'can be seen to have set the stage for our modern conceptions of the elderly as a group that is a burden to society'.[25] Over the course of the century, as Ottaway reveals, the aged themselves were beginning to be more easily defined as a separable group according to their calendar ages, and, she argues, more identifiable as a dependent portion in society.[26] Bolstering this new sense of group identity, as Botelho points out, was England's growing cash and credit-based economy. The development of annuity schemes allowed the wealthier members of society to spend their final years in what we would recognize today as 'retirement': a concept 'fundamentally unknown before'. The elderly, Botelho claims, were increasingly aware of themselves as a social group with needs of their own, and found themselves particularly well-positioned to take advantage of the emergent medical and consumer culture.

Ottaway's work is based predominantly on quantitative historical analysis: censuses, parish registers, family reconstitutions, wills and Poor Law account books. As such she has provided an excellent quantitative framework for exploring the more body-centric and identity-centric aspect of aging in eighteenth-century England. This book takes a different, although complementary, approach to the work that has been done by historians of old age and aging, for it considers 'aging' not as a stage of life – old age – but as a process. Its subject is the essential and epistemological nature of changes experienced, how past societies have set about defining them, and the parameters they set for managing them. As such this work provides an intersection between the work done on aging from a socio-cultural perspective, a history of the eighteenth-century body and a history of identity.

Identity and the Body

In the historical discipline, body studies owes its greatest debt to the poststructuralist enterprise of Michel Foucault. Foucault drew attention to the fundamental distinction between nature and culture. He stressed the power of culture to create the experience of being human, especially the experience of the body. His work emphasized the inevitable constructedness of apparently 'natural' aspects of human experience, and demonstrated how bodies may be involuntarily subjected to systems of power through (particularly medical) discourse. In terms of history, Foucault suggested that the Western body as we know it came about on the back of a profound paradigm shift. This occurred with the advent of 'biology' at the end of the eighteenth-century: the new science apparently coined by Reinhold Treviranus (1776–1837), professor of mathematics and medicine at the University of Bremen. With the advent of biology an entirely new way of looking at and understanding the body was made possible. The 'body' was to be anatomically perceived, professionally defined and scrutinized by a new 'medicalized' gaze. Agency and authority over the body passed from the individual to the medical establishment.[27] Since the influence of Foucault was felt in the historical discipline in the early 1980s, histories of the body have been frequently concerned with mapping distinctions between nature and culture, particularly with regards to the advent of recognizably 'modern' conceptions of bodiliness.[28] In the Foucauldian scheme, the eighteenth century presents a transition period: an era en route to biology and modernity.

As historians we are now familiar with the idea that the 'self', the 'person' and various other mechanisms for comprehending identity, are historically-specific concepts that all have their own history. Identity concepts are created by contingent world views; social, cultural, legal and political trends. Thanks to the legacy of the sociologist Marcel Mauss, we now have a particular narrative that explains how earlier and alternative notions of personhood developed into our modern notion of interior, conscious, psychic 'selves'. Crucially, the development of the recognizably modern 'self' is said to have occurred at the end of the seventeenth century, largely thanks to the philosophical works of John Locke. Consequently, the eighteenth century is also seen as an important gateway between old and new in terms of personal identity theory. Academics from various disciplines have embarked upon the search for the modern self in various social, political, cultural, medical and scientific realms; and charted the rise of the individual in many and various discourses and practices. This has spawned an impressive historiography – one that would be impossible to summarize briefly here. Since it pertains most directly to my final chapter on age and identity formations, the reader will find the story of the coming of the modern 'self' related at the beginning of Chapter 6.

When it comes to the history of categories of identity like race, class or gender, mapping the relative balance of nature and culture been the foundation stone for historical analysis. And in relating the history of embodied identity, the eighteenth-century is said to have witnessed a paradigm shift. Historians have put various aspects of identity under the microscope: gender, sexuality, race and class. Dror Wahrman, in his compendious *The Making of the Modern Self; Identity and Culture in Eighteenth-Century England* (2004), set out to be as inclusive as possible, even considering the distinction between humans and animals. Yet there is nothing in his study – or indeed any other study to the best of my knowledge – about age as identity. This project hopes to cast some light on whether it is possible to think about age and aging in this way, and whether such a narrative applies in the history of aging. To date in the historical discipline we have been somewhat over reliant on thinking about aspects of identity as being rather static. Adding age to the mix draws attention to the inherent mutability of identity concepts, and indeed to the protean nature of human identity itself. It is not my assumption that age and aging are identity concepts that can be deconstructed in the same ways as race, class or gender. Still, this work suggests that adding age and aging to the historian's toolkit can shed new light on eighteenth-century subjectivities. By so doing, we acquire a new lens for looking at the various categories that make up our notions of who we are.

Medical Advice and the Medical Culture of Eighteenth-Century England

Ideas about aging and aging bodies can be found in many disparate places in eighteenth-century England. It would be possible to write a history of aging from a number of different historiographical standpoints. My specific endeavour is to investigate how aging was known and represented through print. This work considers the aging body as a medical, social and cultural construction, and as such it examines historical sources that represent the aging body in prescriptive ways rather than how it 'really was'. Primarily I consider the books that offered literate, health-conscious consumers routes to health and longevity; books which described to them the mechanisms of their aging bodies, and which suggested the ways in which they could be managed. Included within these parameters are medical texts, longevity texts, medical advice literature and textbook physiology. Yet the printed sources that helped make up the medico-consumer culture of eighteenth-century England are multifarious and unclassifiable. Some of the works consulted are relatively well known to us as historians, such as George Cheyne's *Guide to Health and Long Life* of 1724 or William Buchan's *Domestic Medicine* of 1769. Others are more obscure. In addition to works that might be defined as broadly 'medical', I consider a number of works concerned with body matters and psychosomatic self-control. Finally, in seeking to work at an epistemological level, I have found it necessary to consider ideas from a variety of founts in order to build the fullest overall picture possible. This has involved looking at dictionaries and encyclopaedia, conduct works, periodicals, poetry, ballads and devotional works. Although separated by tone, content and form, are united by their interest in age and aging.

The physical body loomed large in eighteenth-century consumer society: it had social currency, a great visual immediacy; it was a fashionable commodity to be shaped and performed. Physical identity became all the more exigent as the ownership of looking glasses increased.[29] Fascination with matters corporeal manifested itself in a desire to discipline the body through dieting and deportment: bodily management became a matter of social responsibility.[30] Yet this was a culture also fascinated by corporeality and its exciting, wayward caprice. Issues to do with the distinction between representation and reality, surface and depth found expression in many divergent discourses and practices: in the new consumer culture of health, in the work of physicians, philosophers, novelists and insurers; in the practice of politeness and the 'cult' of sensibility; in the obsession with theatrics and the sensation of the masquerade.

Self-control and corporeal management played an important role in constructing and legitimating forms of socially acceptable behaviour. Refined discipline of the body was central to the construction of 'politeness', that amorphous concept which, as Lawrence Klein notes, has come to represent 'attentiveness to form, sociability, improvement, worldliness and gentility'.[31] Politeness was a social phenomenon, an art of sociable interaction concerned with integration and 'pleasing' in company. The undeniable importance of bodily management in this cultural regime is confirmed by the 'high density' of medical insertions in the *Gentleman's Magazine*. The most successful of all eighteenth-century monthly periodicals – founded in 1731 and with a circulation touching 10,000 – the *Gentleman's Magazine* was an unfailing barometer of 'polite' taste and reflected the concerns of middle-class consumers. As Roy Porter has shown, within its pages elite practitioners sent items of medical interest, medical books were listed and reviewed, case histories appeared, and readers would write in expectantly with their own complaints, consequently receiving remedies and advice.[32] A demonstrable interest in good health, hygiene and body management was in itself a reflection of the new, polite aesthetic.

Printed advice was the fulcrum of this commercialized, body-centred, self-fashioning medical culture. Advice manuals, describing at once how the body worked and how to manage it were the instruction manuals for this hopeful, careful regime. The genre of 'medical advice' literature considered here consists of proscriptive treatises and manuals aimed at an educated, but definitely lay reading public. Written by physicians – men in receipt of a medical education and in theory privy to the latest scientific and physiological developments – these works do not simply mete out advice, but also provide quite sophisticated descriptions of how the body works, and how treatments brought about their effects beneath the skin. As such, these works may also be seen as a kind of lay physiology, for it was through such material that the body and its subcutaneous mechanisms might be 'known'.

Medical advice literature is all about self-control; it is by nature an empowering discourse, concerned with the relationship between man as rational self-conscious agent and his material body. It has its own attendant form: medical advice speaks to the self-interested reader and tells them what might be done; they presume interested activity on the part of the reader. Medical advice literature is a dialogue between those who knew, and those who wanted to. The genre was not confined to a specialist market of readers, but it was certainly not for everyone. The market itself was somewhat self-determining; those who bought health manuals bought into a cultural aesthetic, for purchasing medical advice was an act of self-definition which marked the buyer as a fashionable health consumer. It was not always a priority for authors to define the ages of their imagined readers, or even what constituted 'old age' in their eyes. Rather, they considered their advice applicable from middle age onwards: Cheyne's observation that 'every Man past Forty is either a *Fool* or a *Physician*' was oft repeated.[33] Writers often explicitly appealed to the virtues of taking care of oneself, and sometimes they spoke particularly to those who imagined themselves most vulnerable. Cheyne, who authored the seminal *Essay on Health and Long Life* (1724), identified his readership in the preface to the work. For high livers and hedonists the book probably held little interest, he thought. However, it could offer real pearls of wisdom to those who sought health, hope and solace via the careful management of their bodies. As Cheyne explained,

> the Robust, the Luxurious, the Pot-Companions, the Loose, and the Abandoned, here have no Business, their Time is not yet come. But the Sickly and the Aged, the Studious and the Sedentary, Persons of weak Nerves, and the Gentlemen of learned Professions, I hope, by the divine Blessing on the following Treatise, may be enabled to follow their Studies and Professions with greater Security and Application, and yet preserve their Health and Freedom of Spirits more entire and to a longer Date.[34]

The advice within medical literature was not readily or specifically gendered, but from the innumerable references to 'old men' and 'old men's healths' one could conclude that the imagined reader was male, educated and probably nearing the decline of life. On the other hand, Cheyne's works in particular appealed to a particularly 'sensible' market: one that was inclusive, both in terms of age and sex. Whereas Marie Mulvey Roberts has interpreted Enlightenment interest in combating aging and extending life as an overtly male and rational endeavour, it should be noted that by the mid-eighteenth century, as George Sebastian Rousseau points out, there were a number of books concerned with health and bodily management aimed exclusively at women. For example, the *Female Physician* of 1739 was reprinted many times.[35]

Medical advice was not a new genre. Cheap works with broadly medical themes had been available throughout the sixteenth and seventeenth-centuries, and from the mid-seventeenth century onwards there had been a veritable explosion of vernacular medical books. The 'marked increase' in medical writings that occurred in eighteenth-century England was a Europe-wide phenomenon, and reflects a more general growth in all types of printed matter over the course of the century.[36] However, it was in the eighteenth century that medical advice had its real heyday: it became recognizably more authoritative, up to date and scientific. Whereas in the sixteenth and seventeenth centuries, cheap books 'hastily compiled by greedy booksellers', often 'poorly printed' and 'written in atrocious English' had flooded the market, the medical advice of the eighteenth century was authored directly by physicians rather than Grub Street hacks.[37] Hence, medical advice was part of a long tradition of affordable, commercially produced and lucrative vernacular health writing, and also part of a new commercially and culturally driven enterprise centred on 'popularizing', rationalizing and domesticating medicine.

For Porter, it was the democratizing impetus that was to characterize and differentiate the medical culture of eighteenth-century England. The spread of printed health manuals was 'crucial' in 'supplanting a traditional, quasi-magical oral health culture with simplified versions of elite medicine'.[38] Yet we should not overestimate the novelty, or 'modernity' of eighteenth-century medical advice. From a modern perspective, the content of some of these works will seem anything but scientific or rigorously medical. Ideas in medical advice constitute a veritable mixture of old mantra, folklorist remedies and progressive physiology. An early work from 1691, *The Way to Health, Long Life and Happiness*, combined advice on temperate living with guidance on children, herbs, fleas and marriages.[39] Even as late as 1819, Dr Trusler's health and longevity guide devoted considerable space to discussing tea, snuff and personal beauty.[40]

Most importantly, it was in this newly commercialized climate of publishing and popularization that the *aging* body became a fashionable site for management and a target for commercialized, prescriptive enterprises. Although promises of 'long life' and 'health' sat together intuitively, twinned in the titles of medical literature since its inception, 'prolongevity' was now seized upon with alacrity. 'Prolongevity' is a term that was coined by Gerald Gruman in his 1966 article on the history of life extension in philosophical discourse, and refers to the significant extension of life by human action.[41] Although the question of whether man could (or should) extend his lifespan was a time-honoured philosophical and theological conundrum, it was during the eighteenth century that potential life-extension enjoyed greater exposure in public culture.[42] Prolongevity became a marketable commodity and circulated in the new mass of affordable print, culminating in a cultural phenomenon that Marie Mulvey Roberts has described as the 'commercialisation of life extension'.[43] Not only pervasive in print, life extension – not to thousands of years, but certainly beyond the sixty or so that one might expect to reach in eighteenth-century England – also had a tangible, visible presence: in the ready supply and demand of purportedly life-prolonging treatments, diets and remedies thrust at a consumer society by physicians and quacks alike. As it was advertised, hawked, discussed, and practised, prolongevity introduced the concept and its attendant issues to a wider audience, calling into question the very meaning and value of aging as something to be managed and controlled.

Prolongevity was a significant plank in Enlightenment philosophy; a tool for discussing man in his socio-political realm. For the first time in the history of ideas about life extension, belief in progress outweighed most of the apologists who had claimed it was neither desirable nor possible, and the extension of human life came to be discussed as a conceivable goal for the future. Enlightened ideas of progress and the perfectibility of man as a social animal blended easily with ideas about prolongevity, finding their apogee of expression in the closing decades of the century, when even immortality was mooted as possible. As Mulvey Roberts explains,

> the notion of mortality as a curable condition may be regarded as an ultimate threshold of Enlightenment meliorism ... [it] represented a secular version of spiritual immortality, a barometer of progress, a world where scientific advances could improve on nature, or, in the light of Godwinian ethical prolongevity, would evolve from socio-political reform.[44]

It was because prolongevity was so intrinsically linked to health, and man's potential influence over it, that it had such mileage for the consumer society of the eighteenth century. The careful management of health and regimen had historically been championed as the route to longevity, with the enduring legacies of mediaeval and Renaissance writers confirming that in order to gain long life one had to live a temperate one. The idea of a long life, and an easy, good old age as reward for physical temperance and moral integrity was deeply entrenched. In the eighteenth century, prolongevity theses intersected with and helped shape a simultaneous snowballing interest in dieting and regimen, the disciplining of the body, and a secularized culture of death and its preparations. Health and prolongevity were mutually supportive: a promise of life extension could be a useful tag line for any commodity addressing itself to the preservation of health. The 'commercialization of life extension' allowed the previously theoretical question of whether or not man could extend his life to be exposed to and absorbed into day-to-day material culture. It allowed the literate or semi-literate consuming public greater scope to consider the length of their own lives, and to consider the boundaries of life and time as finite (or infinite) concepts. As the subject of life extension permeated, it must have mingled with and provoked other questions and ideas about the meaning and value of growing old, youth and age. Aging and the aging body became more visible, potentially more problematic, but also more intriguing.

There is perhaps no better figurehead for the medicalized, rationalized, polite and sensible culture of eighteenth-century England than the famous 'fat doctor', George Cheyne. His *Essay* was a contemporary favourite and has since been hailed by historians as a forerunner of geriatric medicine.[45] As a practitioner in the fashionable spa town of Bath, Cheyne wrote for, and mixed with, the literati and upwardly mobile who suffered lifestyle diseases like the Gout. Those who sought his advice included Robert Walpole, Samuel Richardson, Samuel Johnson and perhaps David Hume.[46] Cheyne therefore wrote about bodies of the historical moment, feeling the strains of luxury in a newly commercial and sexualized society. In fact, Cheyne had his own brush with hedonism in early life, ballooning to a spectacular thirty-two stone after an extended period of indulgence, and then embarking on a punishing regime of somatic and spiritual reform. He famously described his own nervous collapse in his autobiographical 'case of the author', which he appended to his 1733 treatise *The English Malady*. Healing the body through rigorous diet and the mind by religious devotion was Cheyne's combined and mutually re-enforcing philosophy. The *Essay of Health and Long Life* was a perfect example of this combination of practical advice and moral exhortation.

Yet as conservative and traditional as such advice might seem, this came from a man of progressive scientific principles. Cheyne was one of the key proponents of a new system of medicine informed by Newtonian natural philosophy. By 1702 he had been elected as a fellow of the Royal Society and established himself as one of the most prominent of Newton's acolytes there. The desire to expose the complex workings of the body to his readership is manifest in his works; as Anita Guerrini has shown, his recommendation of white meats and vegetables was illustrated through a detailed analysis of their efficacy in Newtonian idiom of attracting particles.[47] Cheyne has proved an enduring subject of attention for scholars, who emphasize the multi-dimensionality of his works, and indeed the man himself. The figure of Cheyne embodies so many elements of eighteenth-century culture. He is at once doctor, patient, scientist, pietistst, asceticist, glutton, autobiographer, commercial entrepreneur, popularist and Man of Feeling. As David Shuttleton argues, his work must be seen as a key part of 'an emergent psycho-therapeutic discourse of middle-class literary consumption'.[48]

The 'remarkable aspect' of Cheyne's career, according to G. S. Rousseau, was 'the uncanny way in which he engaged the public's attention'.[49] His unprecedented weight loss recounted in the *Essay* was vociferously 'consumed' by the public, and his books allowed him to sustain a readership enjoyed by few other authors of the day – medical or otherwise. Both Cheyne and his publishers reaped vast profits from the reprints and reissues of his *Essay* and his later work, *The English Malady*. Yet not all the works considered here were authored by men with anything like Cheyne's kudos, nor did they necessarily share his philosophical or physiological principles. Although written in the same year as Cheyne's *Essay*, Sir John Floyer's *Medicina Gerocomica* differed immensely in tone and content. *Medicina Gerocomica* was one of the few eighteenth-century works dedicated exclusively to health in old age, and is exceptional because of its subscription to Galenic physiology – an idiom that was going out of fashion by the 1720s. Floyer, a Lichfield physician who counted the young Samuel Johnson among his patients, published over ten medical works in both English and Latin, demonstrating an ability to write suitably turgid texts for the medical market, and more accessible health manuals for the more popular one. *Medicina Gerocomica: or The Galenic Art of Preserving Old Mens Healths* was a vernacular text, intelligent, densely written and not 'popular' in comparison with the works of Cheyne. However, it went through several editions, and others of Floyer's works earned him a considerable reputation. Like his more famous contemporary, Floyer's works are underwritten by rationalizing, democratic impetus, an impetus that reached its apex in his promotion of cold bathing and support for charitable construction of chilly public baths.

Ultimately though, it was the populist, contemporary and colloquial tone of Cheyne and his straightforward *Essay* which was to inspire the majority of medical advice works in this period. Another of his contemporaries was the London physician and translator of the works of Boerhaave, Edward Strother. Strother made explicit reference to the teachings of Cheyne in the titles of his own medical guides, which were also named in a somewhat derivative fashion. It was Cheyne's avocation of pious abstention that earned him an important devotee outside the medical profession: the father of Methodism, John Wesley. Relying heavily on Cheyne's oeuvre, Wesley wrote his own popular health guide, *Primitive Physick*, in 1747. It was this best-selling manual that brought Cheyne's medical aphorisms to a wider audience, and continued, through its incredible popularity, to do so until the end of the eighteenth century.

Health and longevity were not topics confined to medical men. Writings about the aging body in eighteenth-century England were as likely to be penned by ministers as they were by medics. The Nonconformist minister Richard Steele's *Discourse on Old Age* (1688) was something of a seminal text, broaching medical and philosophical as well as strictly devotional issues. Conversely, physicians who wrote about the aging body diversified their output. As well as writing two guides on health in later life, the notorious and prolific physician John Hill (1714–75) published on the Gout, insects, botany, gardening, plays, married life, Greek and Roman classics, and dramatic works and fiction based on his having trained as an actor.[50] His oeuvre was remarkably diffuse even by eighteenth-century standards: he published ninety-six books with twenty-nine different publishers during his lifetime. Hill was producing works of natural philosophy from the 1740s onwards, including *Thoughts Concerning God and Nature, the Useful Family Herbal* and *The Construction of the Nerves*. His two titles which considered the phenomenon of the aging body were *The Old Man's Guide to Health and Longer Life: with Rules for Diet, Exercise, and Physick* (1750) and *The Virtues of Sage, in Lengthening Human life: with Rules to Attain Old Age in Health and Cheerfulness,* (1763). Both works went through at least five editions. We should not integrate Hill's polymathy as amateurishness; in fact he corresponded with the great physiologist Albrecht von Haller and included simplified (although essentially correct) synthesis of Haller's works in his own health guides.

It does appear that the topic of longevity was one that had a certain sensational draw, for it inspired no small number of outlandish theories. Later in the century the subject attracted the attention of another eccentric polymath, Philip Thicknesse. His *Valetudinarians Bath Guide: or, The Means of Obtaining Long Life and Health* of 1780 considered how to go about achieving longevity by inhaling the breath of attractive young ladies of Bath. 'I am myself turned sixty ... yet, having always partaken of the breath of young women whenever they lay in my way, I feel none of those infirmities which so often strike my eyes and ears in this great city', he boasted.[51] The breath theory had been mooted in a medical satire in the 1740s. The German doctor Johann Heinrich Cohausen's popular *Hermippus Redidivus, of the Sage's Triumph over Old Age and the Grave* had actually proved the theory in terms of contemporary chemical medicine. Perhaps the most eccentric of all was the physician-magician James Graham, the 'high priest of health and prophet of prolongevity'.[52] Earth bathing, sexual electro-therapy and fasting were among Graham's proffered treatments for aging and mortality, and he communicated his ideas through several publications in the 1790s. Many more titles were authored by obscure or even anonymous physicians. No trace remains of the Dr Bernard Lynch whose *Guide to Health Through the Various Stages of Life* went through several editions in the mid-1740s. Collections might well include 'long life' in their title as a positive selling point. *The Nurse's Guide, or The Right Method of Bringing up Children* (1729) penned by an 'Eminent Physician', for example, promised its readers a bonus 'essay on preserving health and prolonging life'.

Some health and longevity titles enjoyed great commercial success and became the century's bestsellers. Cheyne's *Essay* was an enduring classic going through seven editions in the first year, a further fourteen editions in the next fifteen, and was still in print a century later. Wesley's *Primitive Physick* ran to twenty-four editions by the end of the century. By far the bestselling of all was *Domestic Medicine*, by the Edinburgh physician William Buchan. The book cost six shillings (not sufficiently cheap to be bought by labouring classes, but affordable for the full range of middling sorts), and the five thousand copies initially printed in 1769 sold out rapidly. It remained in print for over ninety years and was one of the most widely owned books in eighteenth-century England. Before the twentieth century, no single health guide enjoyed as much popularity. There were 142 separate English language editions between 1769 and 1871.

As John Mullan puts it, *the raison d'etre* of writers like Cheyne, Wesley and Buchan was education, social improvement and 'popularization'.[53] An assured tone of empowerment resonates through these texts. The core message of Cheyne's *Essay* was that bodily management was the responsibility of the individual. In his opening pages, he explained how, despite the need for soliciting conventional physic in curing diseases, the obtaining and maintaining of health was certainly within the realms of possibility for 'the far greatest Part of Mankind'. Once the internal mechanics of the body could be known – and here Cheyne could empower his readership by describing them – health could be achieved through regulation of the forces of nature. As Cheyne put it, 'The Means are mostly in our own Power'. Buchan stated baldly that, 'most men may enjoy health if they will',[54] with 'proper care' it was entirely possibly to achieve 'an extreme old age', and enjoy 'good health to the very last'.[55] The Scot's work also carried a more radical charge: he denounced the medical profession for its secrecy and mystery, and aimed to 'lay open' medicine to all, by 'shewing people what is in their own power'.[56] In later life Buchan allied his philosophy of medical democracy to the principles declared by the French Revolution, interpreting his research as aiding democratic knowledge and the rights of man.[57]

Mind over Matter

The eighteenth century was the age of new and ready availability of all sorts of lotions and potions. But, as well as this unprecedented use of medicines, the eighteenth century was also an era intrigued by the concept of 'mind over matter' as physic. Interest in psychosomatic therapies had been sparked by increasing anatomical investigation and current developments in natural philosophy: the research of Thomas Willis, René Descartes, Isaac Newton and John Locke, and later the physician-philosopher David Hartley who was to provide the foundations for modern 'psychology'. Consequently, the mind and its 'passions' provided an ever more promising route to understanding, and perhaps mastering, the body and its changes, and by extension, increasing emphasis was placed on psychosomatic routes to health and longevity.

As received wisdom made clear, good health and maximum longevity required proper regulation of the six 'Non-Naturals': food, sleep, evacuations, air, exercise and 'the passions'.[58] Scholars have often equated the eighteenth-century concept of passion as closer to our own notion of 'emotion'. Yet passions were complex psychosomatic experiences, crossing the boundaries between mental and corporeal, spiritual and physical, immaterial and material, conscious and unconscious, external and internal, and cannot be equated with notions of emotion as mental, cognitive entities. As Barbara Duden explains, 'feelings [were] embodied'.[59] Also, unlike our understanding of emotion, which conveys something deeply personal and interiorized, the passions were taxonomic: a set of responses both knowable and classifiable. The business of cataloguing the passions had begun with Aristotle; Aquinas, Descartes and Hume added further and more complex stratifications.[60] In eighteenth-century thought, passions were disruptive experiences capable of deflecting both body and mind from their natural operations and bringing about temporary derangement, disorder or ecstasy. As Descartes had explained in his *Passions of the Soule* (1650), 'noe thoughts shake like the passions doe'.[61]

The leading medical schools of Western Europe were to devote considerable attention to the therapeutic effects of the passions. As the elite physician Alexander Monro mused, 'the doctrine of substituting one passion for another' appeared particularly propitious, and John Lettsom urged the Royal Society to initiate scholarship on the subject.[62] The prestigious Fothergill medal was offered as prize, and was awarded to William Falconer for *A Dissertation on the Influence of the Passions upon Disorders of the Body* (1788). Perhaps the best-known and most comprehensive treatise on what we would now term 'psycho-somatic' medicine was translated into English in 1760. *On the Passions: or A Philosophical Discourse Concerning the Duty and Office of Physicians in the Management and Cure of the Disorders of the Mind*, was the work of the eminent German physician and chemist, Hieronymus David Gaubius (1705–80). The main tenet of Gaubius's work was the utter insuperability of the health of the mind and that of the body. 'Physicians should never keep the body and mind in isolation', he insisted, consequently suggesting that 'physicians ought to be well skilled in philosophy, both as a preparative and as an assistant to their practice.'[63]

Management of the passions was considered of the utmost importance for good health and long life. 'The Passions have a greater Influence upon Health and Long Life, than most People are aware of', Cheyne told his readers sharply, and he devoted a considerable portion of his *Essay* to the subject.[64] In Cheyne's scheme, passions could be regulated by means of diet and attention to spiritual needs; but uncontrolled, they could would wreak havoc on the body via the nervous system. His later work, *The Natural Method of Cureing the Diseases of the Body, and those of the Mind Depending on the Body* (1742), gave fuller exposition to this line of thought. Equally, Buchan's chapter on the passions in *Domestic*

Medicine recognized the value of the passions in therapeutics and suggested that they were ignored at one's peril:

> The passions have great influence both in the cause and cure of diseases. How mind acts upon matter will, in all probability, ever remain a secret. It is sufficient for us to know, that there is established a reciprocal influence betwixt the mental and corporeal parts, and that whatever disorders the one likewise hurts the other.[65]

Managing the aging body could be presented as a psycho-somatic enterprise. As we shall see later, there were even those who thought that aging might best be understood as a case of mind over matter.

Chapter Overview

This book comprises six separable but related chapters, structured thematically. Chapter 1, 'Words and Concepts', goes right back to basics: it is about the very concept of aging itself. What exactly did aging mean in eighteenth-century England, and what ideas might the word convey in the mind of eighteenth-century readers? The chapter investigates eighteenth-century concepts of age and aging by examining contemporary terminology, definitions and linguistic usage across a broad range of sources. It also provides something of a preparatory discussion for the ideas represented in forthcoming chapters, seeking as it does to familiarize the reader with contextual linguistic usage and the semantic potential of the word 'age' in eighteenth-century parlance.

Having considered words and concepts, Chapter 2 considers the aging body and its cosmological significance. The purpose of this chapter is to take a look at the big picture, to provide a wide-angle lens on the subject of the aging body. Why did the body get older? What was the significance of the aging body within the eighteenth-century world view? What did an aging body signify, and what were the conceptual frames with which it might be interpreted? Eighteenth-century people certainly did not look first and foremost to their bodies to understand their aging process; nor could the aging body be understood solely via the researches of science. There were many reasons why bodies were said to change over time, many conceptual frameworks through which the aging body could be understood and interpreted. The chapter takes into account interpretative schemes from various modal levels: the social, spiritual, cosmological and physical. In so doing it draws attention to the great breadth of significance occupied by the aging body in the eighteenth-century imagination.

From this big picture we zoom inwards dramatically, moving from macrocosm to microcosm: we look beneath the skin. Using an approach that is typical for histories of science and philosophy, Chapter 3 considers the impact of a new physiological paradigm and its impact on conceptions of and presentations of the aging body. In particular it considers how this dominant model of physiological function – the 'hydraulic mechanism' coined by Herman Boerhaave and the sensible body that it spawned – enabled writers to envisage the possibilities for human agency over physical aging. The chapter debates the ways in which mechanism presented a radical epistemic shift in the very concept of aging. It also considers the practical and cultural legacy of the paradigm shift in medical advice literature of eighteenth-century England. I argue that although the aging body had always been presented as a problem to be alleviated in popular health and medical writings, the relationship between aging and agency was presented in new, more assured, more scientific and more psychosomatic ways: ways that allowed the aging body to be identified as a particular site for self-control.

Chapter 4, 'Society and Sociability', examines how the significance of the aging body extended into the realm of the social. The aging body became a site for investigating the forces of society and interactions between people. The concept of 'cheerfulness', I argue, was the lynchpin of this significance. In a medical context, cheerfulness was a particular psychosomatic state that provided an antidote to the aging body, a means of self-preservation against physical and mental decline. Cheerfulness was not only a personal but also a political issue: a moral principle of public virtue. Like sympathy and benevolence, cheerfulness was not just an immaterial state of mind, but also a transferable material quality. It was a means of suggesting how interactions between people were potentially physical rather than purely psychic or spiritual. Due to the unique, historically specific way that the aging body was understood at this time, mastery of the aging body became a social, moral and political project, as well as a way of expressing ideas about human nature and public virtue.

Chapter 5 examines representations of old men in medical advice literature. Although this book considers the aging process rather than old age as a life stage, this chapter breaks the mould by investigating what we can learn about prescriptive behaviour in old age from medical advice. As such, the chapter presents how eighteenth-century physicians often imagined an idealized subject in their books: an 'old man' who demonstrated the characteristics, behaviours and regimen they wished to promote. To date, considerably more attention has been given to the study of aged women than aged men, and hence this chapter goes some way to redress this. Of course, the subject under study here is not so much the experience of old age as the representation and idealization of old age: a specific behavioural code to which readers could aspire. As such the chapter considers this code as one particular representation of 'aged identity' or 'aged masculinity' on offer and juxtaposes it against other contemporary identity constructions.

The final investigation is more discrete, and combines a historical investigation with a methodological one. 'Identity Formations' uses the aging body as a lens to investigate identity concepts in eighteenth-century England. It argues that certain eighteenth-century identity concepts, particularly the notion of the 'person' and the 'character', were heavily informed by notions of aging bodies. Written into eighteenth-century concepts of personhood are ideas about the aging, changing body: a capacity for a fluid, dynamic identity which took its value from the protean, diachronic potential of the body and the changes it experienced through the life course. Contrary to an established historiography that has emphasized the emergence of the 'self' as the hegemonic rubric for representing identity, this chapter argues that investigating identity concepts from an age perspective highlights the persistence of emphatically 'pre-modern' ways of comprehending identity in eighteenth-century England.

I use part of the concluding chapter to discuss how we as historians can work with 'aging' or 'the aging body' as a tool of historical analysis in the pursuit of knowledge. Finally, I suggest that the eighteenth-century idea of aging presented in this work is not merely a historically specific vision, but one that resembles some of the ideas about aging emerging from current scholarship and research on aging. In many ways, the eighteenth-century idea of aging is not so very far from theoretical positions that social theorists and gerontologists are developing in academe today, especially as they reconfigure the concept of aging along biosocial lines. Of course, this brings us back to the point with which we opened: that the study of aging in past societies – and an understanding of their historical difference – can help us ask more productive and incisive questions about aging in our own.

1 WORDS AND CONCEPTS: THE MEANING OF AGE AND AGING

Introduction

Definition is a central concern in the study of aging, and historical studies of the subject are suitably preoccupied by it. To date, attention has focused exclusively on the definition of old age rather than 'age' itself; in essence, historians have considered how past societies defined 'oldness'. As a consequence, we now know a good deal about the concept of old age in the early modern period.[1] Yet, we have not stopped to explore a more preliminary and fundamental question: what concepts did eighteenth-century people have of 'age' and 'aging'? These are the questions this chapter explores.

Another issue that the present chapter seeks to expose is the methodological influence that gerontology and sociology have exerted on historical scholarship on old age and aging. As stated in the Introduction, much of the history of aging to date has been characterized by investigations into the relative balance of chronological and cultural factors in past definitions of old age. In framing their investigations, scholars resort – seemingly instinctively – to discussing age and aging in terms of chronological versus cultural indicators. Indeed, the chronological/cultural dichotomy has become standard terminological and methodological fare, rather like other nature/culture pairings favoured in cultural history. Susannah Ottaway confirmed this very point in her recent monograph, stating that 'the key feature of nearly all of the research so far completed on old age in [the] pre-modern period is the assertion that old age was defined primarily in terms of physiological attributes rather than calendar years'.[2] Reliance on this bipartite classificatory scheme forms not only the methodological backbone of Ottaway's study, but more importantly it also informs a key chronological narrative within her work: the growing importance of chronological age as a standard of definition. Undoubtedly, this is a crucial narrative in the history of old age, and one that brings it in line with broader narratives of individualization and modernization. Yet, is this historiographical spotlight on chronological age wholly enlightening? Deconstructing concepts along nature/

culture lines is now second nature to us as cultural historians, but in appreciating the heuristic value of this approach we risk trying to understand the past in our own terms rather than those of contemporaries. By framing investigations in this way, historians not only employ modern gerontological terminology, but also use a classificatory distinction that we cannot assume to have existed in eighteenth-century mindsets. Perhaps a better way forward is to try and investigate the words, concepts and schemes that our eighteenth-century forebears used to talk about aging. It is these terms and their meanings that I hope to uncover.[3]

This chapter, then, is about conceptual possibilities. It is based on the premise that patterns of thought are historically specific and determine what may or may not be imagined at any given time. It consists, therefore, of a 'historical epistemology': a quest to expose some of the 'unstructured institutions' that furnish the mind with ideas and shape individuals' understandings of who they are.[4] Methodologically, it is based on the hypothesis that linguistic study may be a productive way to access historically specific modes of thought. In other words, an analysis of contemporary definitions and of words and their contextual usage may provide clues about the particular way in which eighteenth-century people thought about age. What were eighteenth-century writers trying to convey to their readers when they used the terms 'age' and 'aging'? What associations, ideas or visual images might have these words conveyed? Did contemporary writers define these terms, and if so, how? Obviously, this chapter cannot claim to offer an exhaustive survey of eighteenth-century age related concepts. Instead, its aim is to familiarize the reader with those concepts and usages favoured by the writers of the sources consulted in this study. This is not intended to be a genre-orientated discussion, nor does it attempt to locate the origin of concepts within a certain discourse. Instead I demonstrate how ideas are represented and reflected across diverse textual genres. It is my primary concern here to lay down the foundational underpinnings that enable and inform the particular ideas I discuss in following chapters.

Words and Definitions: 'Age' and 'Aging'

We begin with a basic etymological fact: the word 'aging' (or 'ageing') was not in use in eighteenth-century England. The word is not only absent from medical texts, but from dictionaries and encyclopaedia also. Samuel Johnson's *Dictionary* of 1755 provided entries for 'age', 'aged', 'agedly', 'middle-aged' and 'old', but included no recognition of the word 'aging'. This absence highlights several points: one practical, one historiographical–methodological, and one conceptual. In practical terms it means that eighteenth-century writers did not have a convenient term with which to describe a sense of progress through life, or the collective changes that attended it. For example, when the physician Bernard

Lynch wrote his *Guide to Health Through the Various Stages of Life* in 1744, and signalled to his readership that he was about to present a chapter on what we would now recognize as the 'aging' of the body, he had no shorthand phrase at his disposal. Instead, he offered to 'shew' his readers, 'such things as alter our Bodies, and whatever makes them grow old and brings us at last to our Dissolution'.[5] It was possible to talk about 'old age' and its arrival, or 'growing old', but there was as yet no discrete term available to encapsulate the *process* of getting there. There is a methodological conclusion to be drawn here too: our search for eighteenth-century ideas about aging cannot be conducted via a direct linguistic comparison. Indeed, writing about aging in eighteenth-century England is obviously, in a literal sense, a form of anachronism. For simplicity's sake I will continue to use the term – after all, it is far less time consuming than the contemporary expression used by Doctor Lynch – but its use should serve to underline historical difference rather than blind ahistoricism.

The absence of the word 'aging' is telling in rather more significant ways. In eighteenth-century England, there was no specific word to describe (or imagine) a universal human aging process as a concept or episteme in its own right. This is not to suggest that eighteenth-century people lacked ideas about change over time, getting older, or concepts of youth and age. In fact, their frames of reference were both different to ours *and* more extensive; something that will become incrementally more evident in the course of this book. In the remainder of this chapter, in the absence of 'aging', I will consider the meanings and usages of the concept of 'age' in the texts: how it was defined, the ideas it might have conveyed, and how its semantic potential could be employed and exploited.

The term 'aging' may not have existed in the eighteenth-century, but the term 'age', by contrast, was a very full and significant concept. Even today, the word 'age' is semantically complex, and in the eighteenth century, its meanings were just as many and varied. However, there is an important difference between the relative weightings given to the modern and eighteenth-century variations. It is possible to get the gist of this by comparing modern and contemporary dictionaries and encyclopaedia. The current *Oxford English Dictionary* prioritizes the animate and human-centric aspect of 'age': the context in which one might ask, 'how old are you?' Yet in eighteenth-century dictionaries and encyclopaedia, the meaning was rather different. Where we nowadays assume the word to have an inherent human dimension – predominantly we think of age as an aspect of humanity – to eighteenth-century writers, age was not first and foremost a human-centric concept. Let us consider the order in which Samuel Johnson entered definitions for the word in his *Dictionary*.

First of all, Johnson explained that in a primary and basic sense, 'age' could be defined as 'any period of time attributed to something as the whole, or part of its duration'. This is quite straightforward and of course still applies. However, when we progress to examining his subsequent definitions and particularly his examples (of which there were seven in all), the difference between modern and eighteenth-century terms becomes more apparent. Johnson's focus was squarely upon notions of historical time. As he explained, 'age' referred to 'a Succession or generation of men', or, 'the time in which any particular man, or race of men, lived, or shall live'. For clarity he added 'the age of heroes' as an example. For his next definition, Johnson continued to prioritize the historical value of the term. He explained that 'age' connoted a specific length of secular historical time, and that it was to be understood as synonymous with 'the space of an hundred years', or 'a century'. Only in its fifth sense, was 'age' given a human-centric definition, and this was still not that of the modern sense of an individual possessing an 'age' as a fact about themselves. Instead, Johnson explained that 'age' could be understood as an alternative term for 'the latter part of life; old age' or 'oldness'. 'Age', in other words, could be a direct signifier of 'old age', the final stage in the early modern life cycle. Closely related to this definition was Johnson's sixth entry, where he suggested that 'age' might convey a broad sense of 'ripeness'. Finally, Johnson ended his definitions by acknowledging that 'age' had specific legal connotations concerning the age of maturity and consent.

The fifth and sixth definitions outlined by Johnson – the equation of 'age' with old age or oldness – were common in medical advice literature throughout the century. Often, physicians spoke of age rather than old age. For example, John Hill, writing his guides to health and longevity in the 1750s and 1760s, referred to the possibility of dying 'of age'.[6] In a similar sense he remarked that 'labour brings age before its time', and that 'violent passions' and 'intemperance', exacerbated the 'bodily infirmities of age'.[7] The physician John Bethum, writing in the 1770s, cautioned his readers to 'beware' of exchanging the 'passions of *Youth*', for 'those of *Age*'.[8] In other words, 'age' was not only a shorthand term for old age, but also carried inherent associations with the decline of life and its physical and psychological manifestations.

If it is possible to use Johnson's *Dictionary* as a reliable signifier of eighteenth-century parlance, it seems that the meaning of 'age' was not entirely different to our own, but that its key semantic resonance was in the arena of historical rather than personal time. 'Age' was not first and foremost bound up with the idea of human experience; the word was more likely to signify a period of time, or a chunk of history. This reading seems to be confirmed by the nature of the insertions on 'age' in contemporary encyclopaedias. Like Johnson's *Dictionary*, encyclopaedias published throughout the eighteenth century prioritized the chronological, historical, classical and even astronomical value of the word 'age', and definitions involving personal time were presented as of secondary value. Typically, the entry on 'age' in Ephraim Chamber's seminal 1728 *Cyclopaedia* opened without reference to notions of human lifetime at all:

> AGE: A certain portion or part of duration applied to the existence of particular
> objects: thus we say, the age of the world, the age of Rome, &c. that is, the time or
> number of years elapsed since the creation of the world, or the building of Rome. See
> ASTRONOMY, Of the division of time. The ancient poets also divided the duration
> of the world into four ages or periods; the first of which they called the golden age,
> the second the silver age, the third the brazen age, and the fourth the iron ages.[9]

When human age was explicitly the matter under enquiry, the meaning presented was closer to our notions of lifespan or the life cycle, rather than the idea of a specific, quantifiable 'age'. When the *Cyclopaedia* suggested that 'AGE, properly denotes the natural duration of the LIFE of man', this clearly referenced a concept of lifetime as a holistic entity – the potential sum of it. As Mary Dove has explained, in early modern parlance, the term 'the age of man' referred not to the specific age of an individual, but to the very concept of life itself. During the sixteenth and seventeenth centuries it also became synonymous with 'a long time'.[10] As in Johnson's *Dictionary*, the *Cyclopaedia* also explained that the word had specific, quantitative meanings: denoting either one hundred years ('*seculum*'), or thirty years ('*generation*'). An 'age' was therefore a means of measurement of human life, or a term that could convey portion or part of it. It was in this latter sense that it was possible to say one had 'liv'd several ages'.[11]

As all early modern historians are no doubt aware, 'age' was necessarily and implicitly associated with the life cycle – the ubiquitous early modern socio-cultural map of life.[12] As the *Cyclopaedia* confirmed,

> AGE is also understood of a certain state or portion of the ordinary life of man,
> which is divided into four different ages; viz, INFANCY, YOUTH, MANHOOD,
> and OLD AGE.[13]

The semantic potential of the word 'age' to convey life-cycle stages was referenced in the titles of countless medical books and conduct works, and this continued to be the case well into the nineteenth-century. Somewhat confusingly, 'age' could refer to the life cycle as holistic entity, or simply to one particular stage within it.[14] (The 'age' of man could be made up of several different 'ages'.) On the whole, human 'age' was defined predominantly as a window of time within life, and rather than being accounted for in years; it was conceived in 'portions', 'parts' or 'states'. Emphasis lay on the age of men, rather than the age of a man. In sum, eighteenth-century concepts of age (and indeed time itself) stretched beyond the human to the cosmological and historical, and the appreciation and measurement of it could be via discrete windows as well as linear development. To complicate matters, because the term 'age' functioned as shorthand for 'old age', it could be understood as the final 'age' in the life cycle.

Age as Decay

As this section demonstrates, 'age' could be synonymous with disease, degeneration or decay. As such it functioned as a medical term in its own right, signifying ideas not about time, but about the body, and about health. Similarly, the term 'youth' had a particular value as a health concept: not merely representing, but actually signifying health and life in very literal ways.

By today's reckoning, youth is measured temporally while health is measured medically (physiologically or psychologically). However, in eighteenth-century usage, there was far less of a distinction between the two ideas: 'health' and 'youth' were used so interchangeably as to be practically synonymous. For example, when the physician Everard Maynwaringe, author of *The Method and Means of Enjoying Health, Vigour, and Long Life* (1683), set out to define 'health' for his readership, he named it 'that which supports the fragility of a corruptible body; and preserves the verdure, vigour, and beauty of Youth'.[15] When Maynwaringe described preserving youth, strength and beauty he joined the three concepts together as if they were signifiers of the same material phenomenon. Whereas today we might define beauty and strength visually: 'youth', we might say, is a stage of life defined by years. Not so for Maynwaringe: 'youth' here is a visible condition that may be preserved beyond the boundaries of time. In the opening pages of his work he addressed and defined his imagined readers as,

> they that desire to live *long*; to see their Childrens Children; to preserve their *youth*, *strength* and *beauty*; to be free from molesting pains, and loathsom diseases; to preserve their senses, and enjoy their *endowments* of mind, to the *extremity* of Age.[16]

In such contexts, the value of youth and age becomes body centric, as if they are concepts without value on the temporal plane. Youth and age can be discussed as body conditions, and it seems that writers expected their readers to imagine specific body configurations when using these words.

It was also possible possible to talk about the restoration of 'youth' to somebody advanced in years through the restoration of health. Youth was preservable with health, and if health could be preserved into old age, it was possible to be in a state of youth while being (chronologically) old. Consequently, it was even possible to write about 'growing young again'. This specific phrase was employed in a work of 1722. *Long Livers: A Curious History of such Persons of Both Sexes who have Liv'd Several Ages, and Grown Young Again*, attributed to the Grub Street writer and translator Robert Samber, was one of many commercial publications devoted to sensationalizing human longevity. The book opened by meditating on the great age of the patriarchs and 'long livers' in various 'ages' of the world, followed by anecdotal vignettes of centerians in living memory. Claims that such persons had 'grown Young' rested on reported incidents of these old-timers growing new teeth or having hair restored from grey to its previous colour. The idea and format of *Long Livers* was replicated several times later in the century, and subsequent publications included more recent examples of this ostensible rejuvenation. A Venetian consul was famously reputed to have had his hair changed from grey to black after indulging himself in the company of children and young people, and in 1818 a Miss Jane Lewson was reported to have 'cut two new teeth at the age of eighty-seven'.[17] Based on the frequency with which such anecdotes appeared in the literature, it seems that these tales of strange metamorphoses were both common and fascinating among contemporaries, and retained their appeal well into the nineteenth century.

Whether eighteenth-century people believed in these tales or whether any of them actually experienced physical morphosis or teething in senescence is of less interest here than the terms and concepts that could be used to describe them. At the conclusion of *Long Livers*, Samber told his readers that his foregoing anecdotes offered conclusive proof of the possibility of regaining youth. 'These examples prove Rejuvenescency possible', he effused, adding that, 'to grow young again is to re-enter that beautiful Season, which bestows on us all the Agreeableness and Vigour of the most brilliant Youth.'[18] To modern eyes, Samber's claim seems somewhat ludicrous, and of course it is difficult to gauge how literally such claims might be intended or received. What seems likely is that when Samber and others like him suggested that his long livers had 'grown young', he did not necessarily imply the same meaning that this phrase is likely to convey today. What it connoted for Samber (and presumably his readers) was indeed a transformation, but one that was predicated on definitions of 'youth' and 'age' that were interpreted predominantly within the parameters of health and the body. If youth, in an eighteenth-century context, could be understood as a health condition, then it was possible to conceive of growing young in a similar way that one might make a recovery of health after a period of illness, or as the result of particularly beneficial regimen. Seen in such terms, ideas about growing young no longer appear linguistically problematic, nor conceptually so strange and alien. It was possible therefore in eighteenth-century England to talk of growing young as well as growing old.

The understanding of 'age' as a disease with visible symptoms and functional impairments dated from antiquity. It was Galen who first described old age as a natural disease. The main textual source that familiarized eighteenth-century readers with this idea was written by the thirteenth-century philosopher and Franciscan friar, Roger Bacon. His original work, *De Retardatione Accidentium Senectutum*, was translated in 1683 by the physician Richard Browne under the title *The Cure of Old Age, and Preservation of Youth*. Browne's translation remained in print throughout the eighteenth century, and other fragmentary translations appeared, especially in volumes of collected works. Through such works and innumerable references in medical advice, Bacon was established as the primary referent for the notion that old age, or just 'age' was a pathological condition. As Browne explained to readers with sombre glee in the preface to his translation, 'you make every day a considerable step toward Old Age, which is it self a Disease'.[19]

In essence, the work configured aging within the linguistic parameters of disease: age could be diagnosed via various bodily symptoms, and, like a disease it might be treated with various medicinal or therapeutic strategies. What we might nowadays refer to as the 'symptoms' of disease, Bacon termed the 'accidents' of age, and explained that the condition might be diagnosed via their physical manifestation. Bacon was also influential in setting the standards for what the disease of old age looked like, and what those suffering from it might experience. Within the Franciscan's list of 'accidents' were some factors that we continue to associate with aging today, 'grey Hairs', 'Paleness' and 'Wrinkles of the Skin' for example. Yet in addition to these innocuous, cosmetic factors, a host of ostensibly more pathological – and unpleasant – conditions were tabulated, including 'Diminution of Blood and Spirits, Bleareyendess, abundance of rotten Phlegm, filthy Spitting, Shortness of Breath, Anger, Want of Sleep' and 'an unquiet Mind'.[20] These latter issues appear explicitly psychological to the modern eye, and quite removed from the notion that 'natural' aging may be quite gentle and benign. In formalizing a recognizable 'disease', of age, Bacon undoubtedly forged a conceptual link between 'age' and unpleasantness. He had certainly set the tone for configuring the concept if not in medical terms then certainly in terms of health and the body, disease and decay.

However, because age could be understood as a disease, something isolatable and autonomous, it might be treated, or even cured. Within Bacon's seminal scheme, treating age was not a case of retarding a process, but of attending to specific 'accidents'. In fact, because the disease was known and defined through its accidents, removing them could remove the sufferer from the condition itself. The accidents of age, Bacon explained, might be 'taken away'.[21] Moreover, it seems that Bacon thought it possible to enter and exit the condition of age in a way comparable to the experience of and recovery from disease. Correct manipulation of these accidents facilitated a removal from the condition of age and possibly even an extended experience of the condition of youth. 'All hot Oyls preserve Youth', he stated, 'so far as they hinder the Falling and Greyness of the Hair.'[22] Just as a subject might be diagnosed ill or well, it was possible to conceive of being within the condition of age. Once the symptoms were removed, the condition would be alleviated or cured.

The conceptual synonymy between age and decay is at the heart of one of the key discourses on aging available in the eighteenth-century England. *A Discourse Concerning Old-Age, tending to the Instruction, Caution and Comfort of Aged Persons*, written in 1688 by the Nonconformist minister Richard Steele, was a widely sold work that went through eighteen editions and remained in print for the first half of the eighteenth century. Steele authored several works of popular piety, and the *Discourse*, which aimed to assist those facing their last years to obtain religious certainty, is ostensibly a devotional work. Still, Steele's remit in writing the *Discourse* went beyond the demands of popular devotional literature in its contemplation of philosophical and physiological issues. A glance at its tabulated contents serves to demonstrate the significance of aging in various realms beyond the strictly spiritual. Working at something of an epistemological level, he sought actively to define and explain the 'Nature' and the 'Causes' of aging, as well as comment upon its attendant virtues, vices, comforts and privations.[23] The *Discourse* is particularly important for our purposes here because of the lengths that Steele went to in defining his concepts of 'age' and 'old age'.

In his opening sentences, Steele made a conscious stab at semantic deconstruction for the benefit of his readers. He began by telling them that first and foremost it was necessary to conceive of 'Man's *Age*' as a concept consisting of three autonomous portions. 'Man's *Age*', he wrote, 'seems most fitly to be distributed into 1. His *Growing*. 2. His *Ripe* or consistent, and 3. His *Decaying* Age'.[24] It was on this last stage or 'age' that the treatise was focussed. 'And so we are come to the *Third* and *Last* Stage of Life, the *Decaying* Age or *Old-age*', wrote Steele, explaining that this was 'namely, *The Part of Mans life, wherein through the Multitude of Years his Strength is decay'd*'.[25] It was crucial for Steele to explain to his readers that technically, old age was a result of both time and decay. It was 'not *merely* such a *number* of Years without some *Decay* of Nature, that can properly denominate *Old-age*', he reasoned. 'Neither ... doth the *Decay* of *Strength* alone, determine a man Old':

> *Diseases* and other Casualties may weaken and wither him, who in respect of his Age, hath not attain'd the *Meridian* of his Life ... But when our *Strength* is decayed through the multitude of *Years,* then *Old-age* commenceth[26]

As if this needed further clarification, Steele went on to affirm that,

> from whence it followeth, that neither *Gray-hairs,* nor *Wrinkles,* nor any such separable *Adjunct* can be a Demonstration of *Old-age;* seeing Sickness, or Cares, or Fears, or Grief may produce these Effects, without a considerable Decay of strength, or Number of years ... Thus *Authors* tell us of those, whose Hairs have become *hoary* by *Sickness,* and have grown black again at the return of Health ... But all these being preternatural and accidental, do not constitute Old age at all.[27]

Whereas Steele offered a distinction between the effects of disease and the effects of time, he made an implicit recognition of the conceptual proximity of these ideas. He noted that '*Diseases* and other Casualties' may weaken a subject at any stage of life, and suggested that grey hairs and wrinkles are often the product of 'Sickness, or Cares, or Fears, or Grief' rather than old age. Essentially he acknowledged that both types of decay might look the same. We are left wondering exactly how possible it would have been to distinguish between the two, especially in a society with far less access to medical or cosmetic treatments. For all his specificity, Steele appears to imply that old age and disease are visually insuperable, and that the very same notion of 'decay' is the central and definitive characteristic of both.

Bizarrely (for the modern reader at least), Steele states that being advanced in years did not constitute old age: it was 'not *merely* such a *number* of Years without some *Decay* of Nature, that can properly denominate *Old-age*', he claimed. It seems rather strange to think that a person might be chronologically old and still not qualify for 'old age'. Yet for Steele, this is entirely conceivable. In order to be old, or to be in the state of old age, it was absolutely necessary to be decayed. It was impossible for Steele to conceive of old age without 'decay'. Not surprisingly, therefore, when considering explicitly whether old age might be defined chronologically, Steele was adamant that it could not:

> Now touching the precise *Year* wherein Old-age may be said to begin, it is not so *material* to be known, as it is *doubtful* to be fixed ... It's true, an universal *fixed* period cannot be set herein; the diversity of mens natural Constitutions, Imployments, Diet, Exercises, *&c* causeth Old-age to come *sooner* to some, and *slower* to others.[28]

In this extract, it seems that 'decay' is not considered solely attendant on the passage of time, but is something autonomous, like a disease. Old age may be understood as an event or bodily condition, the arrival of which may be known via various symptoms manifest on the physical body. Steele's definitions point to the real proximity of 'age' and 'decay', conceptually and physically. His difficulty in separating them, the linguistic porosity and their shared symptoms suggest at least the potential for conceptual congruence. The boundaries between concepts of age and concepts of disease in eighteenth-century England must have been at least indistinct, and perhaps at times invisible.

Even at the end of the eighteenth century, it was possible to imagine old age as a pathological condition. This sentiment was given an explicit airing by the German doctor, Christoph Hufeland. Hufeland was something of a latter-day George Cheyne, a practising physician with clients among the literati, the most famous of whom were Schiller and Goethe. His *Art of Prolonging Life*, written in 1794 and translated into English in 1796, promoted a new science of life-prolongation that he termed 'macrobiotics'.[29] His extensive study consisted of an analysis of various practices that were either detrimental to or helpful towards the prolongation of healthy life, and it offers a critique of various current social and personal behaviours and practices. In an early condemnation of the unhealthy living conditions in industrial cities, Hufeland identified and vilified the practice of 'ingrafting' old age 'on youth':[30]

> We may see at present, particularly in great cities, men come to maturity in their eighth year; in their sixteenth, attain to the highest point possible of their perfection;

in their twentieth, struggling with every infirmity, a proof that they are already on the decline; and in their thirtieth, have every appearance of exhausted age, such as wrinkles, dryness and stiffness of the joints, a crooked spine, loss of sight and memory, grey hair, and a tremulous voice. But it is not enough that people now attain old age, in a period during which our ancestors were still young: they unfortunately go farther. They have found out the art of bringing into the world children with old age upon them. Such phenomena I have sometimes seen. These shriveled beings enter upon the stage of life with the strongest features of age; and, after two weeks spent amidst misery and crying, they close their aged life, or rather begin existence by ending it. But I shall draw a veil over these horrid productions of parental dissipation, which appear to me like the embodied sins of the parents.[31]

Leaving aside the sentiments here, it is clear that the concept of old age may be used (albeit rhetorically) to suggest a state of bodily decay which is, as Hufeland makes quite explicit, independent of any sense of age in a chronological context. Indeed, in Hufeland's extract, even children may display 'the strongest features of age'. The 'age' or 'old age' that Hufeland describes here is – like those of the thirteenth-century Franciscan, and the late seventeenth-century minister – a disease, bodily decay, the embodiment of malignity and corruption. It is a factor that, like disease, may be brought about by living conditions and especially by poverty. Although Hufeland's motive above is undoubtedly a moralizing one, the language he uses is testament to the semantic power of the word 'age' to convey concepts and images of decay to the eighteenth-century reader. Whether couched in pseudo-medical terms, as pathology, or as the embodiment of social corruption, the very word 'age' had a particular and distinctive meaning: the potential to directly convey a certain malignity.

A Language of Opposites

The ability to comprehend age as a disease, and more specifically the tendency to juxtapose this condition against 'health' or 'youth', may be understood as an example of what Stuart Clark has identified as 'binary thinking'.[32] As Clark explains, the human tendency to revert to dual classifications – the primeval opposition between good and bad – has been in evidence throughout discourse since Aristotle. By the sixteenth and seventeenth centuries, the 'predisposition to see things in terms of binary opposition' was 'a distinctive aspect of a prevailing mentality'.[33] Clark finds a 'remarkable frequency with which the 'language of contrariety' was called upon to standardize arguments and notes its extraordinary pervasiveness in early modern discourse. To Clark it is clear that audiences and readers were able and expected to make sense of their world in these ways. Certainly this is in evidence in discourse about youth and age in the eighteenth century, and nowhere is it more obvious than in the literature of humour or polemic.

This section briefly demonstrates the use of this rhetorical device in both conduct literature and the myriad of popular printed material about 'May and December' marriages. The subject of age-disparate marriages was an attractive subject for eighteenth-century moralizers and jeremiahs. Deliberation over the virtues and vices of age-disparate marriages was a common feature of early modern conduct literature, and the subject was a well-established and enduring topic of poems, plays, jokes and ballads.[34] This is hardly surprising given that considerations of age in conduct literature nearly always pertained to the issue of fertility. For, as Daniel Defoe explained in his, *Conjugal Lewdness: or Matrimonial Whoredom* (1727), 'the principal End of Matrimony' was 'for the lawful Procreation of Children'.[35] For the most part, conduct writers advocated a 'sacred condition of equality' between partners, which meant a desirable similarity of social status and age.[36]

Since the fertility span experienced by men and women in the eighteenth century was akin to that of today, technically this opened up the possibility of marriage partners being quite disparate in years. Legally, men and women were considered to have 'Natural and Corporal Ability to perform the duty of Marriage' at fourteen and twelve years respectively.[37] The menopause brought the end of women's fertility between the ages of forty-five and fifty, and in exceptional cases, as Defoe noted, 'Men ... had Children at a very great Age'. When it came to marriage, as Keith Thomas noted, at least some disparity in age between marriage partners was 'very common', whether the older partner was male or female.[38] Not surprisingly, marriages between older women and younger men attracted a disproportionate amount of attention. However, such unions were a reality as well as mere fictive fodder or patriarchal paranoia, and had long provided young men with a recognized mode of advancement. Conduct writers focused their attention on decrying marriages with the greatest disproportion of age. This could be for the purposes of venting anxiety, self-righteous morality, or just plain amusement.

The stereotypes of youth and age were well-worn characters, particularly in the vocabulary of satire, where they had an enduring appeal.[39] The predatory older woman (frequently a widow) and the young man intent on fortune hunting were familiar caricatures, as was the impotent old lecher. The youth/age dichotomy had a long-standing appeal, and it would be facile to suggest that it isn't an irresistible rhetorical device with a lot of imaginary potential. However, it is not so much remarkable that youth and age could be set up as oppositional in these texts, but rather that this youth/age duality was integral to shaping the arguments themselves: age could be used as a standard of explanation in its own right. George Booth, author of *The Present State of Matrimony: or, The Real Causes of Conjugal Infidelity and Unhappy Marriages* (1739), envisaged youth and age as diametrically opposed conditions. Booth's own tempestuous marriage – as the penniless Earl of Warrington he was compelled to marry a rich heiress – induced him to publish the jeremiad advocating divorce on the grounds of incompatibility of temper. Bemoaning the 'present state of matrimony', he included youth and age on a list of well-worn good/bad opposites where youth was implicitly associated with beauty, innocence and health, and age with deformity, debauchery, diseases and rottenness:

> In short, we see Beauty coupled to Deformity, Youth to Age, Innocency to Debauchery, Health to Diseases and Rottenness; that we may as well join Fire and Water, War and Peace, and all the Contraries in Nature, and expect a reasonable Result from them, as expect any solid Happiness in innumerable modern Marriages.[40]

Setting youth and age into a list of 'categorical sets through which we live and make sense of the world' was to suggest that they were fundamentally, naturally different.[41] As Booth would have it, the opposition between youth and age was one of the 'contraries in Nature', one of the pairs of binary opposites long entrenched in the early modern imagination. The 'natural' disjunction between youth and age had also been emphasized by the late seventeenth-century health and conduct writer, Thomas Tryon, in his *The Way to Health, Long Life and Happiness*. 'When Young and Old intermarry', he wrote,

> there is an inward, natural, and therefore unappeasable contrariety, loathing and dislike between them, whence ariseth Aversion, Hatred, Jealousie, and Irreconcilable Discords.[42]

Similar sentiments and sense-making strategies surfaced in the anonymously published *Batchelor's Monitor* of 1743. Therein, the youth/age disjunction was conceptually insuperable from a canon of other 'natural' oppositions: lightness/darkness, summer/winter: the various cosmological binaries evoked ubiquitously in the early modern world. Indeed other pairs of opposites were called upon to emphasize the significance of the youth/age disjunction:

> For what can be more unnatural and preposterous, than to go about to unite brisk and sprightly Youth with dull and senseless Age? They might as well have undertaken to have joined Summer and Winter, Light to Darkness, or any other such likely Piece of Business, as to think with all the Strength of Imagination to couple together a young lusty Piece of Flesh with an old frigid Statue.[43]

In this reading of age concepts, youth and age were fundamentally, naturally different. 'Age' in this context was loaded with meaning a state of decay, the negative 'other' to youth.[44] The marriage of youth and age was not merely the marriage of two people of disparate years, or where disparate years signalled or suggested disjunction, it was (explicitly) the union of opposing conditions, and therefore doomed. Differences in age between people could be presented as differences of kind rather than degree. Far removed from a modern understanding of aging as a continuum, youth and age were imagined here as independent concepts – opposites.

Of course, that the eighteenth-century mindset was attuned to working with binary sense-making schemes is evident in a number of cultural practices involving the body. As Roy Porter observed, the eighteenth-century body and its 'paraphernalia of movements, expressions and garments' was invested with 'a universal sign-grammar of good and bad'. The power of juxtaposition, inversion and stereotyping was evident in the vogue for Theophrastan 'characters', physiognomy and – the cultural form famous for its 'logic of symbolic inversion' – the masquerade.[45] The satirist Edward Ward, in composing his *The Amorous Bugbears: or, The Humours of a Masquerade* (1725), described in this poem the covert liberties afforded to those trapped in age-disparate marriages via the camouflage of this subversive social gathering. In so doing, Ward took the opportunity to capitalize on the semantic potential of the terms 'youth' and 'age', contrasting 'old Beldams' with concepts of 'Strength and Health', and aligning 'age' with impotence and disease:

> Some, in the zenith of their Strength and Health,
> Match'd to old Beldams for the sake of Wealth,
> Among the Crowd steal hither to refresh
> Their wanton Appetites with younger Flesh,
> That they the pleasing difference may tast,
> 'Twixt Parchment-Udders and a tender Breast.
> Some Dames by Parents in their Youth betray'd
> To warm old Misers, in the fruitless Bed
> Of Age and Impotence, where nothing dwells
> But teasing Coughs, dull Groans, and sickly Smells,
> Mix also with the rest, in hopes their Charms
> May tempt the vig'rous to their craving Arms[46]

In such contexts, use of the terms 'youth' and 'age' signify images of flesh in extreme states of health: vigorous youth and decrepit, impotent old age. Here, as in many similar examples, age concepts have a particular value: the power to signify visually. Thanks to innumerable instances of this linguistic trope in poems, ballads and moralizing texts, eighteenth-century consumers would surely be in no doubt about what 'age' looked like.

Although this has been a linguistic analysis, clearly it would be misguided to ignore the content and context of this textual material. Concerns about age disparities could help articulate a host of other anxieties about possible disruptions to the relationship between husband and wife, or operate as a weapon against the perceived corruption in society. Writers who attacked the over-sprightly elderly often wished to pour scorn on the market forces which indulged luxury and allowed 'Sir Courtly' figures the cosmetic trickeries to conceal their withering bodies. Such tirades can never be isolated from a broader concern that aimed at stigmatizing the decadence and profanity of the upper classes, or mocking the social aspirations of middling consumers. It seems at least that the ability to construct youth and age as polar opposites was a useful device for driving home arguments and anxieties. These devices had a particular force because they relied on 'age' to signify iniquity, corruption and decay.

Conclusion

This chapter set out to investigate eighteenth-century concepts of age and aging by examining contemporary terminology, definitions and linguistic usage. The analysis has focused closely upon texts that offer either specific definitions or extended and explicit discussions of the terms in question. It has drawn attention to a particular and historically specific facet of the eighteenth-century concept of 'age' that was striking if not paramount in popular conduct and medical literature, and has also pointed to some rhetorical contexts where use of this particular concept might be especially salient. As such, the ideas represented here are considered illustrative of those represented in the body of literature discussed throughout the course of this book, and their characteristic nature will become increasingly apparent as the reader progresses.

In the eighteenth century 'age' had a broad field of reference – it referred to time, the cosmos and history as well as humanity. The ubiquity of the life cycle as a sense-making scheme ensured that aging could be interpreted as sequential states or stages. 'Age' also had a particular power: the ability to signify concepts of disease and decay. Although we might expect to find concepts of age and aging that prioritized health and the body in medical advice literature, the point to be gleaned here is not that health writers focused on body-centric elements of aging, but that the very term 'age' could by itself convey pathology, decay and corruption. Since Bacon, if not Galen, it was possible to imagine old age as a disease, indeed to call it a disease in specific terms. However, arguably this was less of a 'disease' in the modern sense of geriatric pathology, and more of a nebulous, metaphysical, abstract concept of 'decay' in a very powerful, perennial and cosmological sense. It was this kind of universal iniquity and degeneracy that the term 'age' could be called upon to represent in conduct literature and popular print. And as such, 'age' could be used as a standard of explanation in itself: illustrating ideas about polarities, extremes and opposites, and about the distinction between good and bad. This conceptual configuration could be put to powerful rhetorical or polemical ends in both didactic and humorous contexts.

In very broad terms, the findings in this chapter suggest that eighteenth-century people thought about aging within the conceptual parameters of health and the body as opposed to those of time and individual diachronic development.

Of course, when put in these terms, this corresponds with the historiographical consensus on old age. Scholars have agreed that throughout the early modern period old age was measured and defined through predominantly cultural rather than chronological indices. Yet, as this chapter has shown, the issue might be explained at a more fundamental, epistemological level; and in terms that are not merely about old age, but about age itself. It was not just old age, but the bigger, broader concept of 'age' that could be defined with reference to decay. If we accept the potential synonymy between 'age' and 'decay', it seems inevitable that the parameters for framing ideas about age and aging would be those of health and the body and not those of time or years. When seen from this angle, there is little surprise that the visible, functional indicators of old age would be prioritized over chronological ones.

At the beginning of the chapter, we asked whether the gerontological distinction between 'chronological' and 'cultural' age was a useful tool of historical analysis. It seems that, in the contexts examined, this classificatory binary scheme is far less enlightening than the particular binary scheme evoked by eighteenth-century writers themselves: the fundamental, cosmological distinction between good and bad, embodied through notions of health and decay. By now it hardly needs stating that eighteenth-century writers did not employ the terms 'chronological' or 'cultural' age; nor did such distinctions emerge in dictionaries and encyclopaedia of the time. This simple fact forces us to acknowledge that the terms we work with as historians are themselves products of a modern mindset informed by the specific twentieth-century discipline of gerontology.

It is not only modern gerontological terminology that has pervaded historical research into old age. Modern socio-political concerns about an aging population have also been heavily influential in framing historical problems. Perhaps the near obsession with standards of definition has come about as a result of the unmissable visibility of an aging demographic in Western Europe in the twenty and twenty-first centuries. An aging population presents problems of definition for the state and its apparatus. How is oldness to be defined? What is a pensionable age? Should the parameters of old age be redrawn to accommodate population changes? With these socio-political issues come attendant cultural shifts and practices: the emergence of a potentially rich 'grey market' in marketing and advertising, the promotion in the media of the new 'sexy seniors'.[47] In short, in the twenty-first century we are steeped in awareness that aging presents some kind of 'problem to be solved'.[48] It is a phenomenon that seemingly requires definition and control, and perhaps we turn to the past with these thoughts very much at hand, wondering how eighteenth-century people defined and classified the 'old' in society. Ultimately, the nature of our own concerns is highly historically specific. Although it is entirely inevitable that present issues consciously or subconsciously shape historical enquiry, it does seem that a focus on these concerns, particularly modern classificatory schemes, has obscured other and perhaps more basic lines of investigation in the history of aging to date.

We also began investigation in this chapter by revealing the absence of 'aging' in eighteenth-century discourse. Without our concept of 'aging', how did eighteenth-century writers explain how and why the body changed and got older? How did physicians and their contemporaries, whose words we have been analysing, explain the 'aging' of the body to their readers? What were those 'things' that 'alter[ed]' the body in the eighteenth-century imagination? Eighteenth-century people may not have had a particular shorthand term to use, but one word – one master narrative of decline – would not have done justice to understanding the forces of aging in the eighteenth-century imagination. This absence of 'aging' has brought us to the fringes of a big, conceptual, cosmological scheme, and this is the subject of the following chapter.

2 THE FORCES OF AGING: MACROCOSM AND MICROCOSM

Introduction

In eighteenth-century England, it would have been impossible to explain the aging of the body by looking beneath the skin. In the medical imagination and beyond, the aging of the body was seen to happen just as much from the outside in as inside out. Aging involved the imprint of various external phenomena upon the material body. Through an analysis of the texts responsible for describing the aging body to the reading public, this chapter demonstrates that aging was not just a matter of flesh and blood; when it came to interpreting body changes over the life course, medical writers – even progressive medical theorists – did not necessarily look to the body itself for a locus of causation. The physical changes we now associate with aging were understood as matters social, spiritual, moral, historical and cosmological.

Whereas an accepted historiography has highlighted the growing internal, secular and biological significance of the body in the eighteenth century, aging was an aspect of corporeality that was notably resistant to the forces of modernity. The legacy of Max Weber and Marcel Gauchet has ensured that the late seventeenth and eighteenth centuries are seen as a period characterized by the gradual disconnection of the celestial and terrestrial orders and consequent 'disenchantment of the world'. Broadly speaking, bodies could now be investigated as independent entities, subject to their own internal rules and laws; a practice that culminated in the eventual advent of 'biology' at the beginning of the nineteenth century. Historical body studies, influenced by a broadly Foucauldian narrative, have tended to emphasize the growing biological status of the body throughout this period; indeed, the history of the eighteenth-century body has been largely, in the words of Nancy Leys Stepan, the history of 'the *ontologising via embodiment*' of human experience and human identity.[1] Since the early 1980s, histories of the body have been chiefly concerned with charting the rise of this recognizably 'modern' conception of bodiliness.[2] Modern bodies, we are told, were characterized by their inward focus, autonomy and biologically determined nature. Although his overarching narrative has been questioned since, it is Thomas Laqueur who is credited with first explaining how, during the eighteenth century 'the framework in which the natural and the social could be clearly distinguished came into being'.[3] Revisionist scholarship has tended to reposition Laqueur's perceived transition at an earlier date, but few studies have questioned the more fundamental proposition that the eighteenth-century body was subject to a broadly secularizing, modernizing gaze, a gaze that looked inwards rather than outwards.

Although much attention has focused on gendered bodies, this modernizing and biologizing narrative is certainly not to be understood as a story exclusively about 'making sex'. For as Laqueur explained, the 'discovery of the natural body as the gold standard for social discourse' was 'not just a story about gender', but 'part of what would be a more comprehensive history of exclusive biological categories in relation to culture'.[4] As yet we have no particular study that has considered the aging body in this light, and the findings in this chapter offer perspectives on this debate. In contrast to historical scholarship that emphasized how attention apparently turned inwards to comprehend the body on its own terms, this chapter argues that it was still impossible to comprehend the eighteenth-century aging body without reference to a grand cosmological scheme. Nor could 'aging' yet be understood as an exclusively secular issue. Despite the undeniable presence of various 'disenchanting' forces, the old world order that Barbara Duden has felicitously described as the 'Great Code' was an enduring and pre-eminent interpretative framework for the aging body throughout the eighteenth century.[5]

In the previous chapter we considered words and concepts. We move now to considering the perceived causes of aging: the forces that made bodies grow old in the eighteenth-century imagination. There were many reasons why bodies were said to change over time, and many independent interpretative frameworks through which to understand and interpret aging. Each of the following sections deals with a different interpretative perspective. Although each of these factors is considered discretely, I wish to emphasize from the outset how such a set of beliefs and conceptual frameworks were both interrelated and mutually re-enforcing.

The Life Cycle

Historians have long been aware of the significance of the life cycle in early modern thought: it was the mental map, providing a means of interpreting and giving significance to life's experience. Throughout the eighteenth century, as Susannah Ottaway has demonstrated, it remained the central framework for thinking and talking about life. 'People who lived in the eighteenth century ordered their lives by stages', she states. 'Even if they were not aware of their precise chronological age in years, they were aware of their basic position in the life cycle.'[6] The eighteenth century inherited many ways of dividing up life into stages: Aristotle had suggested there were three stages; Galen and Hippocrates said four; Ptolemy seven; the Middle Ages left a variety of models; and Shakespeare had written of seven acts. Within this imagined life experience, childhood, youth and old age were placed in various stages of dependence on adulthood, mirroring pre-industrial society's economic, political and social structure, and complementing the transmission of property and skill from generation to generation. As a transformative point in the life cycle, marriage was the gateway to full, participatory adult life, and the fact of being married or unmarried was one of the main ways of perceiving and representing differences between people.

Etymologically and literally, one's 'age' in eighteenth-century England referred to one's position in the life cycle. Throughout the early modern period, and well into the nineteenth century, the structure and rationale behind conduct works and medical advice reflected the ubiquity of the life cycle as a predominant concept for making sense of life's changes, both societal and physical. *The Female Aegis: or, The Duties of Women from Childhood to Old Age*, published in 1798, shared its ideological framework with that of Hannah Woolley's, *Gentlewoman's Companion ... from Childhood down to Old Age*, written more than a century before. Each organized its advice around what was considered appropriate for the different stages or ages of life, with discrete chapters devoted to each stage.

It is absolutely crucial to understand that the life cycle was no mere abstract interpretative framework. Although rites of passage may now be understood as societal mechanisms, life cycle changes were traditionally considered to have physical effects on those who passed through them. In the words of Laura Gowing, 'age, marital status and social position had tangible effects on the body'.[7] Despite the existence of an established scholarship on the early modern life cycle, considerably less attention has been focused on the real transformative power accorded to rites of passage over the body, or how these apparently abstracted notions were said to 'work' beneath the skin. Historians such as Gowing have undoubtedly recognized the affinity of the life cycle with humoral visions of body function, but some of the more obscure ideas about cosmology and numerology, astrology and aging have been somewhat neglected. The following section looks briefly at these forces and their continued significance in eighteenth-century texts.

Climacteric Years

In the eighteenth century, the powers at large in the cosmos were understood to exert influences upon the human form, and this was especially the case for the aging body. Whereas it is generally accepted that the importance of astrology declined with the advent of the 'scientific revolution', we must not ignore the continued acceptance – or at least the legacy – of some of its more accessible doctrines. One tenet that showed particular resilience was the notion of 'climacteric' or 'climacterical' years. Combined in this precept were ideas about planets, numbers, matter and the human body, and it exerted a considerable influence on explanations as to how and why humans aged as they did.

Given that there were seven known planets in cosmos, the number seven had long been accorded an extraordinary significance in the cosmological schema. Loosely connected to this basic concept was the more general and pervasive belief that ages divisible by seven were invested with great moment. Hence in human life, every seventh year constituted a 'climacteric'. These 'climacteric' years were, rather like the life cycle, rites of passage. The early ones – seven, fourteen and twenty one – signalled legal maturity; the later ones were said to be periods of particular mortality, when the body was in a state of heightened peril. There were two critical years in life: the 'Climacteric Year', which was forty-nine years (seven sevens), and the 'Grand Climacteric Year', which was sixty-three (nine sevens). On top of this (and somewhat confusingly) was the schema of 'enneatic' years, within which every ninth year might prove dangerous or significant.[8] Enneatic years, as Rob Ralley has conceded, exerted considerably less power in the early modern imagination, and drew considerably less scientific or philosophical attention. However, the two doctrines of climacteric and enneatic years combined to reinforce awareness that the sixty-third year of a person's life held particular momentousness, being a multiple of both seven and nine.

Ralley has exposed the complex ideological and philosophical reasoning that supported these theories. Despite ubiquitous references to climacteric years in the early modern period, their meaning was contested and multifarious. Some writers linked them to the movements of heavenly bodies, others, including Thomas Browne (who translated Bacon's discourse on old age) thought that astrological considerations were less significant than the 'extraordinary power and secret vertue conceived to attend these numbers'.[9] Some writers thought climacteric years required a medical explanation: every seven years humours might gather and stagnate in the body. Not surprisingly, the connection between climacteric years and the life cycle or 'ages' of man was, as Ralley explains, 'a standard one for those who covered the topic', and enabled writers to 'draw broader observations than simply medical ones' about the tangible power of seemingly abstract rites of passage over the physical body.[10]

Climacteric years held a position of extraordinary power in the early modern imagination because the doctrine made sense within various streams of thought: ancient, biblical, astrological and medical, not to mention its congruence within the all-pervasive framework of the life cycle. Although Ralley's study does not extend to the eighteenth century, it seems that belief in the basic existence and power of climactericals was enduring. As he concludes, at the close of the seventeenth century, the patterns of climacteric years, and the dangers that attended them, were common knowledge. The astrologer John Partridge (1644–1715) could remark in 1697 that the doctrine was 'grown so commonly known among the Vulgar; that there was not "a Plowman" who could not recite its details'.[11] As Michael Stolberg has pointed out in his study of menopause in early modern medicine, the simple belief that more people perished or became ill in their forty-ninth, or sixty-third years persisted well into the eighteenth century.[12]

References to climacteric years appear in many eighteenth-century texts about the aging body. They are, moreover, accorded a special power to age and change the corporeal frame. Such citations are usually broad references and no more; they are not typically followed by analysis or attribution. Still, a basic awareness of climacteric doctrines (broadly understood) seems to have been at least present in the minds of many of those who wrote of the aging body. Glancing references suggest that readers were supposed to understand the meaning and significance of the term. Take for example one of the most popular Classical texts on old age often cited in the eighteenth century (and very popular in translation throughout) Cicero's *De Senectute* (44 BC). It was said to be composed, as numerous readers would be made aware as they encountered the work, during the author's '*grand Climacteric,* which was the Year before his Death'.[13] An extended reference to the doctrine of climacteric years appeared in a popular ode to the famous centarian, Thomas Parr (of whom more later), where it was suggested that the 'climacterical' doctrine was not only a 'learn'd' and presumably respectable one, but also something 'held in general':

> Amongst the learn'd, 'tis held in general,
> That every seventh year's climacterical,
> And dang'rous to man's life, and that they be
> Most perilous, at th'age of sixty-three,
> Which is, nine climactericals.[14]

Moreover, climacteric years featured in medical texts, and could even be called upon to account for physical change. In Bernard Lynch's *Guide to Health through the Various Stage of Life*, written in 1744, body changes are attributed to the 'Excellency' and 'Perfection' of the 'Number *Seven*'. Lynch opened his *Guide* with the following statement:

> As our Bodies are subject to Changes and Alterations, from the Minute we come into the World; so the *Physicians* ... have divided Man's Life into several Periods, which they call *Ages* ... The *Pythagoreans* ... have publish'd in their Writings, that we undergo remarkable Changes every seven Years, as well in regard to the Temperature of the Body, as the Qualities of the Soul; all which must be referr'd to the Excellency and Perfection of the Number *Seven*.[15]

As this extract suggests, configuring the aging body in eighteenth-century England involved intermingling various ideas about bodies, changes, stages, ages, classical legacies, septennial accounting, body temperature and spiritual development. All are thrust together and seen as ideas mutually reinforcing. For Lynch, aging can be reduced to the special significance of septennial numerology. Although such explicit and fervent attributions are rare, explicit reference to climacteric years did not have to be made for writers to express some concern that particular years held a certain significance for the aging body. As Edward Strother, in his *Family Companion for Health*, wrote in 1729,

> take great care of your Healths, especially about the fortieth Year, for if you are seiz'd at that Time with any grievous Diseases, you will have much ado to escape: this is a Season, when the Fibres grow rigid and the Blood gross and hot; Diseases must then be lasting and vigorous; Consumptions at this Age are very dangerous, because the Humours are now extremely sharp and corrosive; there are some Parts of our Blood, which we have retain'd from our Infancy, and this must of Course be very sharp; at this Season therefore all Caution must be us'd: we must not use too much Exercise, we must feed on smooth and soft Liquors and victuals. This is the Age that most Men dye at … and shou'd we venture a Mistake of Consequence at this Age to the forty-fifth Year, we may depend upon it, it is equal to the Hazard of our Life. [16]

Although Strother's exact numerical accounting does not appear to be in perfect synch with the strict doctrines of the climacteric, he is adamant that certain 'Seasons' in life bring about a real state of physical vulnerability. He even went as far as to suggest that there was empirical evidence on the matter, and encouraged his readers to check the available statistics. 'The Bills of Mortality, which you may read, do testify this Truth', he stressed.[17] These opinions, we should note, were not those of an eccentric astrologer. These were the words of the physician who translated the works of Herman Boerhaave, physiologist, father of material mechanism and venerable man of 'science'. Strother was no stranger to 'new' ideas. Yet, new ideas enabled by paradigmatic changes in physiology were not necessarily seen as incompatible with climacteric ones. Even Boerhaave himself made reference to 'the great Climacteric Year, namely, the sixty-third', in his masterwork of physiology, the *Institutiones*.[18] George Cheyne's *Essay on Health and Long Life* – a text that has been identified as a forerunner of geriatric medicine – is not without references to the climacteric doctrine. In the *Essay*, Cheyne made explicit reference to the climacteric, and suggested that it had affective physical power over the body. It was exactly at the time of 'the great *Crise* or *Climacteric* of Life', wrote Cheyne, that the body was triggered to change:

> Then it is, that the Blood and the Juices of the most Healthy and Strong begin to *cool*, to *thicken*, to become *vapid*, and to be *obstructed* in the *Capillaries* and *Lymphatics;* many of which Vessels, by such *Obstructions,* coalesce and become *cartilaginous,* the *Perspiration* is lessened, all the several *Secretions* are rendered less *perfect*, all the *Solids* grow stiff and hard, and lose their *Elasticity*, and the *Circulation* is gradually reduced

into a narrower Compass, approaching still nearer and nearer to the *Trunks* of the Blood-vessels, or their first Branches.[19]

Sophisticated physiological descriptions, themselves based upon distinctly 'scientific' notions such as the circulation of the blood and the vascular system, could be allied with ideas about cosmology or numerology with no apparent incongruity.

The notion of the climacteric and its real, tangible influence on the body is a difficult concept to fathom from twenty-first-century positions. What seems so radical about such views is that the body is seen to respond to abstract rites of passage and the mysterious, unquantifiable influence of certain numbers. The belief belongs to a mindset that has long since disappeared, and so today we intuitively interpret such beliefs as antithetical to, and therefore incompatible with 'medical' or 'scientific' ideas. However, the fact that such references endured well into the eighteenth century, and moreover that they appear in medical texts, suggests that belief in these powers might transcend paradigm shifts. The persistence of climacteric years is not only remarkable in itself, but it serves to illustrate how ideas about aging were an integral part of a great cosmological schema.

The Christian Tradition

The Christian tradition provided a significant and inescapable frame of interpretation for the aging body. It must be remembered that 'life' in the eighteenth century was not just a journey from cradle to grave, but preparation for the afterlife too. One's experience of aging could be a signifier of moral and spiritual probity; the relative ease or discomfort therein might be interpreted as dependent upon antecedent behaviours and conduct. The twelfth chapter of Ecclesiastes offered the ultimate showcase for a good old age, and many eighteenth-century texts paraphrased its mantra. Richard Steele directed his readers thither in his *Discourse Concerning Old-Age*, noting that '*Old Age* is describ'd in the twelfth Chapter of *Ecclesiastes*, under so beautiful an *Allegory*, that nothing can excel it.'[20] As Pat Thane reminds us, representations of old age in philosophical, theological and even medical texts are as often metaphorical as literal. Such texts may carry a didactic impulse, and Thane is keen to remind us that contemporary texts and images do not necessarily represent old age 'as it was'.[21]

Still, it was possible to interpret body changes as responsive to moral and spiritual thoughts and actions. In the biblical tradition, physical decay was synonymous with both individual and social corruption. Technically, aging was not inherent to humanity, but 'superinduced' as a punishment after the Fall.[22] The link between physical decline and mortal sin was underlined in Steele's *Discourse Concerning Old-Age*. Steele discussed the physical manifestations of aging in some detail, and in doing so he emphasized the idea that their fundamental origin was spiritual. Although Steele defined the 'Natural Cause' of old age as 'Driness and Coldness' – a (humoral) body issue – he located the 'Original Cause' of this physical change in 'Mans sin'.[23] Decay, a central tenet in Steele's definition of age itself, was essentially the embodiment of both the sins of the individual and of mankind. Consequently, spiritual probity could be understood as a counterbalance to aging itself; He was sure that 'Piety' and 'Sobriety' might offer a tangible preservative effect upon the aging body.[24] Where the aging body was concerned, spiritual and somatic issues blended easily; in a work of popular devotion it was entirely natural to discuss the physical manifestations of aging, for the cause of these physical changes could be understood as ultimately metaphysical, indeed divine.

Consequently, the historian will do well to note that eighteenth-century works on aging do not fall neatly into 'medical' or 'devotional' categories. Just as Steele's discourse was ostensibly devotional but contained physiological discussions, a number of other works embodied the conceptual inseparability of the aging body spiritual and the aging body physical. Thomas Tryon's 1704 *The Knowledge of a Man's Self, the Surest Guide to the True Worship of God*, which appears to be a devotional work, was also, as the subtitle explained, a *Way* to *Long-Life, Health* and *Happiness*. In fact the text opened with an 'Anatomical Description of the Body of Man'. Conversely, moralizing jeremiads could masquerade under the appearance of medical works, as in the case of John Harris's *Divine Physician* of 1709. As this pseudo-physician explained, 'The first means' of long life was 'to avoid Sin in general', as it was the 'occasion of bodily Diseases, and shortness of Life'. Conversely, Harris explained, 'vertuous and regular actions and affections' were said to 'naturally conduce to the health of Body, and length of Life'.[25] Sin, immoderacy and wicked thoughts were still very tangible forces of aging, and in this shared belief medical and devotional literature could coalesce.

Nowhere was the link between spirituality and physiology more overt than in the works (and indeed the person) of George Cheyne. Cheyne was not only a physician but also as a devout moralizer, employing contemporary 'scientific' theory to underscore the spiritual dimension of all matters corporeal (an early work, *Philosophical Principles of Natural Religion* (1705) employed Newtonian natural philosophy to demonstrate God's existence in scientific terms). At the core of his teachings was his unceasing faith that sound body resulted from a soul close to God. As David Shuttleton has demonstrated, Cheyne was able to 'reconcile a post-Cartesian mechanistic account of the body', with 'an overtly anti-Lockean adherence to pietist concepts of innate spiritual principles'.[26] This coupling of science and spirituality so idiosyncratic of Cheyne can be seen as an appropriate characterization of eighteenth-century writings on the aging body. Aging bodies in particular are singled out for spiritual advice. In the writings of Cheyne, it was via discussions of the aging body especially that he could really endorse the link between matters somatic and spiritual, for this was a context in which

Cheyne could translate biblical metaphors into physiological terms. The aging of the body, he explained, constituted a return to (not proverbial but real) dust:

> In old men the bones petrify, the cartilages and tendons turn into bones; and the muscles and Nerves, into cartilages and tendons. And all the solids lose the Elasticity, and turn, in a great measure, into that Earth they are going to be dissolved into.[27]

It was this spiritual–somatic idiom that earned Cheyne his most 'enthusiastic medico-religious disciple', John Wesley.[28] Wesley was so taken with Cheyne's aphorisms that he wrote his own health manual, and lifted much of the content directly from the works of Cheyne. *Primitive Physick: or, An Easy and Natural Method of Curing Most Diseases*, was a book of 'Simple Medicines' for 'poor' and 'plain', written in 1747 becoming one of the bestselling and most widely owned books in eighteenth-century England.[29] In his preface, Wesley confirmed that aging and sickness were to be understood as the embodiment of spiritual corruption. 'When Man came first out of the hands of the great Creator', he wrote, he was 'liable to no Decay.'[30] Disease, aging and death were lumped together as the bodily incarnations of spiritual failure.

In sum, the pervasive influence of the Christian tradition ensured that the eighteenth-century aging body could not yet be a secular issue. An eighteenth-century work on the aging body is as likely to be written by a minister as a medic; and the physician responsible for writing the century's most popular text on the aging body was wholeheartedly committed to interpreting health and long life within spiritual parameters. Underwriting the semantic link between age and decay we encountered in Chapter 1 was the biblical association of aging with punishment for human sin.

Lifespan

We understand that human life is a biological universal with finite boundaries and guaranteed decline. Today we use the concept of 'lifespan' to denominate the length of time (especially the maximum length of time) that humans can live. But eighteenth-century England existed in a time and place before the accepted certainty or institutionalization of this doctrine. In the eighteenth century, time and the body had not entered a schematic or formulated relationship; as yet there was no concept of a biological, universal human lifespan. Biblical teaching reckoned the duration of human life to be highly dependent on historical circumstance. As set down in the Bible, and unquestioned in the tradition of prolongevist writings, humans had lived far longer in the distant past. References to the historical specificity of human lifespan and the great longevity of the patriarchs featured freely in numerous medical advice works throughout the century.

As far as biblical dictum was concerned, humans were created immortal, but took on sin and mortality after the Fall. Within this schema, it was reckoned that lifetime had been reduced to roughly one thousand years by the time of Abraham, further depleted to five hundred after the Flood, and to one hundred and twenty in the time of Moses. Therefore it made sense to suppose that the sixty or so years one could expect to live in the eighteenth century represented a Mosaic lifetime reduced by half. Hence a 'normal' lifespan in the eighteenth century could be legitimized and naturalized via its part in the biblical scheme. The human body itself was still considered a historically specific phenomenon, or, to put it another way, the 'age' of the world dictated the age of its inhabitants.

The absence of a concept of a human lifespan allowed for the persistence of an unquestioning belief in longevity, and indeed superlongevity. Whereas it now appears distinctly naïve to entertain the possibility of living until one hundred and fifty-two, this was neither impossible nor implausible to the eighteenth-century imagination. Indeed, eighteenth-century England witnessed a remarkable interest in the lives and lifestyles of celebrated 'long livers'. The *Index* to the first fifty-six volumes of the *Gentleman's Magazine* notes thirty-eight references to articles or insertions on 'remarkable instances of Age' between 1731 and 1786.[31] A demand for printed anecdotes of longevity remained constant throughout the century, and new examples of nonagenarians and centarians were added continually to the ever-expanding catalogue.

Without a doubt, the most celebrated English 'long liver' was one Thomas Parr, immortalized by the late seventeenth-century 'water' poet John Taylor as 'The Old, Old, Very Old man'.[32] Parr, a humble agricultural labourer from Shropshire, was supposedly 152-years old at the time of his death in 1635. Allegedly, his longevity earned him an invitation to the Royal Court, where he was requested to dance a jig for the King. He died soon after this sensuous onslaught, and his death was chiefly attributed to a 'change of air'. A post-mortem was carried out on Parr's body, and the condition of his vital organs noted with some interest. Although this procedure was carried out by none other than William Harvey (responsible for describing the circulation of the blood), the King's physician saw no reason to question Parr's longevity, even though his report shows he found the body suspiciously well preserved.[33]

Belief in the superlongevity of 'Old Parr' and indeed many other famed centarians showed no signs of halt as the century wore on. As both Keith Thomas and Pat Thane have pointed out, these stories were accepted quite faithfully. 'Only in the nineteenth century', Thomas writes, 'did tough-minded investigators get down to the task of exposing these bogus claims.'[34] Parr was a popular phenomenon, and he was often cited as an example of potential human longevity comparable with that of Mosaic times. Taylor's poem, *The Old, Old, Very Old Man* remained in print until the nineteenth century. Parr was not a lone example of course (a Jane Scrimshaw was hailed as 'The Miracle of Miracles' in a short text of 1711), but merely the most visible manifestation of faith in the pliability and flexibility of the human lifespan. To eighteenth-century readers, Thomas Parr and his kind provided proof of the residual potential for patriarchal longevity inherent in the human body; a reminder of its origin, its history, its Divinity.

Even the most progressive and 'scientific' Enlightenment ideas were underscored by a belief in the historical specificity of the human lifespan. The mid-century longevity theorist Johann Cohausen (who we encountered proposing inhaling the breath of young women) was in no doubt about the inherent flexibility of human life. In order to launch his thesis, Cohausen reminded his readers that there was 'no such Thing, as a settled Term of Life', either understood 'by the Law of Nature', or 'by the express Will of Divine Providence'.[35] Lifespan, he wrote, was entirely a matter of 'Contingency'.[36] And it was not only lifespan that this longevity theorist saw as unfixed and malleable: the aging process was likewise: 'There are no settled Periods in Nature, no inevitable Laws which conjoin weakness and Infirmity with a certain Number of Years.'[37]

It was upon similar fundamental principles that, right at the very end of the eighteenth century, William Godwin in England, and the Marquis de Condorcet in France were to posit theories of potential future human immortality. Even though these definitive Enlightenment projects were emphatically forward-looking, they were premised on a distinctly pre-modern and doctrinal notion of the inherent flexibility of human lifespan. How and when one aged was largely a matter of the world in which one lived.

Humoral Medicine and the Language of Temperature

There was an appropriate medical scheme that worked in conjunction with the Great Code: the humoral medicine elaborated in Antiquity by Galen and Aristotle. Strictly speaking it was a medical schema that was, even at the dawn of the eighteenth century, being rendered defunct by the various currents of the 'scientific revolution'. However, despite the 'hankering after the bare mechanical causes of things' that characterized eighteenth-century science in general, it seems that scientific ideas about the aging body remained resistant to change.[38] In fact, one of the only eighteenth-century medical works devoted entirely to the aging body was written in wholehearted humoral idiom.

From antiquity until the dawn of our period, medicine had been theorized and conducted around the Aristotelian–Galenic synthesis of qualities, elements and humours used in natural philosophy. The four qualities of hot, cold, dry and wet were the primary constituents of the body, and indeed of the world. Within this ideology, disease was said to be caused by an imbalance of the humours; a patients 'temperament' became too hot, too cold, too dry or too wet. Medicine operated on the basis of therapeutic regimen: imbalance was to be rectified by taking a remedy or participating in a practice that offered opposing, balancing qualities.

Aging, in humoral terms, involved the body growing colder, drier and harder. Shifts in body temperature were called upon to explain the physical manifestations of the aging process: dry, wrinkled skin, brittle bones and cold, lean hands and feet were all signifiers of the depleted reserves of heat and moisture in the body. Declining heat was the non-reducible principle that provided the explanation for aging and natural death: the 'Principle Cause', in the words of Roger Bacon.[39] With the decline of this 'natural' or 'innate' heat – a property which bespoke not only literal warmth but spirituality, even 'life' itself – came the decline of life and the consequent visible and functional manifestations. The humoral system could explain age changes via the rubric of the elemental register, and equated heat with physical, vital activity within the body.

Now, despite the fact that humoral ideology was on the wane in medical advice as the century progressed, some of the images and ideas from the old scheme remained current. The image or metaphor of natural heat was obviously a powerful and useful one, for references to this vital property (sometimes referred to as the lamp of life, or the flame of life) persisted in medical advice throughout the century, even if the works otherwise eschewed humoral physiology as a central logic. For Cheyne, a mechanist and Newtonian through and through, 'life' could still be likened to the proverbial candle, and an ideal, natural death described as a 'taper' going out 'for want of Fuel'.[40] Despite insisting that the human body was a 'pneumatico-hydraulic machine', it was still entirely possible for Cohausen to write about the 'Flame of Life', and for Christoph Hufeland in 1794 (although life was a peculiar 'chemico-animal operation') there was still such thing as tangible 'vital power'.[41]

Recent histories of bodily experience have shown that the old humoral scheme was especially durable in the minds and words of eighteenth-century patients. Thanks to studies by Barbara Duden, Severine Pilloud, Micheline Louis-Courvoisier and Philip Reider we can see how patients in eighteenth-century Germany, France and England, respectively, continued to talk about their bodies using words and images from the humoral register.[42] Although none of these studies have considered the aging body in particular, it seems likely that aging was something that leant itself to discussion in humoral terms. Even in medical texts there was a marked tendency towards humoral language and metaphor. The language of temperature (if not the full humoral ideology that went with it) proved remarkably pervasive: heat and moisture just seemed intuitive to explaining the aging process. As one anonymous *Eminent Physician* put it in 1729, "tis very easy to conceive that *Old Age* must be cold and dry'.[43] And as Sir John Floyer explained, 'an old Man's Body is like a Plant dried by the Sun'.[44] Old bodies must have looked cold and dry, and it was the 'old' humoral body that had the language, ideas and power to explain it. At least, the basic link between aging bodies and temperature was a strong and enduring one. It was only in 1758 that the prominent physician Alexander Monro debunked the myth that the insane escaped physical aging on account of their supposed resistance to changes in temperature.[45]

Temperament and Character

As an integral part of the humoral schema, the concept of the temperament – otherwise known as 'habit', 'complexion' or 'constitution' – remained absolutely central in writings about the aging body. As Bernard Lynch explained,

> *Temperament* is that Diversity in the Blood of different Persons, whereby it is apt to fall into some certain Combinations more in one Body than another, whether into *Sanguine, Choler, Phlegm,* or *Melancholy;* from whence persons are said to be of *sanguine, cholerick, phlegmatick, or melancholy Temperament* or Constitution.[46]

Medical works prided themselves on offering advice 'adapted' to different temperaments. An extended description of the 'four grand Qualities' might be a useful starting point for any medical advice work. Although technically the concept of the temperament was part of the Aristotelian–Galenic schema, it endured autonomously outside the realms of its founding ideology, pervading advice literature throughout the century. In the 1750s, the leading physiologist Albrecht von Haller stated that although the notion favoured 'too much of the ancient and particularly the Galenical doctrine', he was in 'no doubt' that there were temperaments. Each person had, as he put it, an 'irrevocable determination to this or that habit or temperament'.[47]

The temperament was not just a means of explaining physiological differences between different people; just as importantly, it was a means of explaining differences between the same person at different stages of their life. The temperament altered as one aged; different stages of life were attended by different temperaments. The two concepts of the life cycle and the temperament were mutually dependent and mutually definitive, as Bernard Lynch implied in his *Guide to Health Through the Various Stages of Life*:

> Man, according to the natural Course of Life, undergoes five remarkable Changes in his *Temperament* and passes five Ages or Periods; that is, *Infancy, Adolescency, Youth, Manhood,* and *Old Age.*[48]

The temperament was in many ways the somatic manifestation of the life cycle. It was via changes in temperament that early modern people might feel and experience the changes attendant on the different 'ages' of life. With these temperate and temperamental changes came different emotional requirements, different needs and different desires. The physician John Bethum, in his *A Short*

View of the Human Faculties and Passions of 1770, explained to his readers that shifting positions in the life cycle was attended by both physical and emotional transformation. 'Guard against the passions to which you are liable by your *Constitution, Temper, Age, Station,* [and] *Outward Circumstances*', he wrote. 'Beware of mistaking the *Change* of passions for the *Conquest* of them, as when the passions of *Youth* are exchanged for those of *Age*.'[49]

In an eighteenth-century context, 'The different *Degrees* and *Changes* of Age' were marked by different physiological configurations, and these different physiological configurations would in turn be responsible for changes in passionate experience.[50] It was necessary therefore to 'guard against the passions to which you are liable by your *Constitution, Temper, Age, Station, Outward Circumstances*'.[51] Temperamental characteristics were considered in sync with transformations in the body. Changes in 'character' always involved physiological and material changes, and physiological changes usually have inevitable 'character' changes attendant upon them. Transformations in temperament involved essential change in body, mind, person and character. In such a conceptual scheme, it was entirely possible – indeed inevitable – to imagine that a person would literally switch characters over the life course. That a person's 'character' might metamorphose with age seemed such a logical and obvious truism, that Gaubius hardly thought it needed acknowledging:

> Is it not a trite and common observation, that men, as they pass through different stages of life, not only alter as to their bodies, but also more especially in their minds? How unlike is the old man to what he was in his youthful days, and the youth to an infant, as to their understanding, reasoning, judgment, memory, inclinations, manners and instincts?[52]

Physiologically, everyone experienced being different characters throughout life as a matter of course. The idea that progress through life was in steps – discrete and significant rites of passage as opposed to steady linear development – placed emphasis on tangible breaks and changes in roles throughout the life cycle. Indeed, the terminology used to discuss life and one's progress through it was hence overtly and explicitly theatrical.[53] The process of aging – or going through the life cycle – was by extension integral to the idea of 'character'. In fact, in eighteenth-century parlance, the whole notion of 'character' implicitly referenced aging, the life cycle and the temperamental changes attendant upon it. This is examined in some detail in Chapter 6.

The need to respect the individual temperament was especially pertinent in advice about aging. Indeed, it was the notion of the temperament that was said to account for the differences in aging between individuals. 'The diversity of mens natural Constitutions, Imployments, Diet, Exercises, *&c* causeth Old-age to come *sooner* to some, and *slower* to others', wrote Richard Steele.[54] Edward

Strother explained that 'the longest-liv'd people' were those 'of moist and warm Habit of Body'.[55] Apparently recounting from his own experience, the anonymous author of the mid-century tirade, *The Folly, Sin, and Danger of Marrying Widows, and Old Women in General*, explained to his readers that it was his estranged wife's 'Constitution' that accounted for her residual youthfulness and voracious sexual appetite:

> My Wife, tho' Sixty-five Years old, still preserved a lusty, warm, and vigorous Constitution, and had not the least aversion to the Pleasures of Youth. But as for me, my Habit of Body was weakly and cold, and the Fretting and Vexation which I daily endured, from the termagant behaviour of my Wife, had worn me to a Skeleton.[56]

The notion of the temperament also helped people measure and define notions of youth and age. In the previous chapter it was suggested that concepts of age were largely constructed via ideas about health and decay. The concept of the temperament was another context in which such ideas rang true. Rather like the lusty wife in the extract above, youth could outlast the passing of time provided the temperament remained 'warm and vigorous'. Lynch made it clear that youth and, particularly oldness, were largely temperamental issues. 'Years', he suggested, could not be 'depended upon' to define '*Youth* and *Old Age*'. Rather, he said,

> we ought rather to regulate ourselves by the *Temperament*, or Nature of our Constitution: for we may call every Man that is *cold* and *dry*, an old Man; there are a great many such at forty, and a great number of young Men at sixty. Some Complexions fail sooner, and others later.[57]

Although the concept of the temperament was comprehensible outside the bounds of the humoral schema, in practice its persistence endorsed the language of temperature. When discussing the different 'ages' or stages of life in bodily terms, writers tended to revert to temperate expressions. 'The last Period of Life', wrote the anonymous *Eminent Physician*, 'when the Temperament, that was before hot and moist, is become cold and dry, is call'd *Old Age*'.[58] When Lynch wrote of 'the different *Degrees* and *Changes* of Age' he referenced to very real conceptions of physical alterations in 'degrees' of body temperature. Arguably, it was still the temperament that allowed eighteenth-century writers (and, one expects, readers) to imagine and particularly to *visualize* body changes over the life course.

Non-naturals

Since the ancients, the various forces of nature responsible for health had collectively been tabulated as the 'Non-naturals'. These were air, food, sleep, exercise, evacuations and emotions. As Steele explained in his *Discourse on Old Age*, the body aged 'originally' because of 'man's sin', it aged 'naturally' because of the declining heat in the body, and 'preternaturally' because of exposure to these six factors.[59] The Non-naturals were the tools of Galenic therapeutics, the means of preserving the requisite homeostasis in the body. They endured as an accepted framework for structuring advice on health throughout the eighteenth century, even for those writers who otherwise eschewed the humoral idiom. Cheyne, for example, stated explicitly the practicability and logicality of ordering the advice in his *Essay* under these different 'heads'.[60]

In applied terms, the Non-naturals were also the typical means of advocating that ethic of abstemious moderation so intuitive to Western Christendom. Regimented abstention – expressed as 'regimen' for short – had always been, and continued to be, the accepted route to a long life and an easy old age. Queen Anne's physician, Sir William Temple, had put it quite simply: the 'common Ingredients' of long life were 'great Temperance, open Air, easy Labour, little Care, Simplicity of Diet, rather Fruits and Plants than Flesh ... And Water'.[61] According to Cheyne it was 'Abstemiousness', that would lay the 'Ground work' for longevity; and William Buchan's 1769 bestseller, *Domestic Medicine* opened by stating that regimen was 'the most valuable part of medicine'.[62] The eighteenth century inherited two epic heroes of regimen: the Belgian Jesuit, Leonardus Lessius (1554–1623), and Luigi Cornaro (*c.* 1468–1566), a Venetian nonagenarian whose masterwork, the *Discorsi della Vita Sobria* claimed that Ciceronian strict temperance – indeed near starvation – was the secret of his longevity. Cornaro in particular received frequent reference in eighteenth-century medical advice, but English translations of the works of both enthusiasts continued to be produced throughout the century, often collated together. The *Discorsi* went through no less than fifty editions in the course of the eighteenth and nineteenth centuries, and Joseph Addison did much to advocate and popularize Cornaro's punishing scheme in the *Spectator*.

The Non-naturals were not only the means by which health and longevity might be achieved. They were also forces directly responsible for aging the body. Eighteenth-century writings on the aging body accorded these forces of nature an extraordinary physical power. On the one hand, the body was seen as extraordinarily vulnerable to these external phenomena. On the other, its readiness to respond to them meant that body management was guaranteed to have predictable – and beneficial – results, founded on perceived compatibility and interactivity between micro and macrocosm.

Visions of transcendence between external and internal worlds are wholeheartedly definitive of the work of Cheyne. For the great fat doctor, essences inside and outside the body were of a piece. In his writings on the aging body, external influences, particularly foodstuffs, were presumed to transfer their essential characteristics to the body, and indeed to the mind. 'The thinner my diet is', he commented, discussing his own reformed proclivities, 'the easier, more cheerful and lightsome I find myself.'[63] When it came to providing advice about the aging body, the key was to eat the kind of food that could provide inherent qualities of suppleness. Properties in the food would be transferred to the body's structure, preventing fibres from becoming hard and inflexible and facilitating a better circulatory principle. Essential qualities in food could be transferred directly to the body – lightness in food created lightness and ease of function, and lightness of mood. Hence, 'the Grand Secret and Sole Mean of Long Life', Cheyne wrote,

> is to keep the Blood and Juices in a due State of Thinness and Fluidity, whereby they may be able to make those Rounds and Circulations through the animals Fibres, wherein Life and Health conflict, with the fewest Rubs and least Resistance that may be ... Tho' the Solids must necessarily harden by old Age, so as to stop the Circulation; yet this may be retarded by keeping the Juices fluid by a meager and diluting Diet.[64]

Body fluids and external fluids could be considered of a piece; a thin and diluting diet was directly compatible with the structures of the body and could have a direct affect upon the quality of the blood. The aging body itself is not seen to be a discrete object; it interacts dynamically with the Non-naturals in the outside world.

Sir John Floyer and his *Medicina Gerocomica*

In eighteenth-century England, there were few medical works devoted entirely and exclusively to the aging body. So it seems quite remarkable and perhaps significant that the most comprehensive, rigorous and 'medical' of these was written in the humoral register, Sir John Floyer's *Medicina Gerocomica, or The Galenic Art of Preserving Old Mens Healths* (1724). This final section of the chapter is devoted to a brief look at Floyer's humoral body-world, for his complex yet elegant scheme is testament to the power of the humoral register to explain and account for physical aging. In particular, his work provides a fascinating insight into the mysterious and hypnotic power accorded to the concept of 'heat' in the old scheme, and why it might be such an indispensable trope for comprehending aging. Floyer shows us a body at the mercy of the outside world, porous and malleable, and in doing so he provides further proof of how, in eighteenth-century England, aging was a phenomenon that could happen from the outside in.

Floyer was a staunch adherent and champion of the Aristotelian–Galenic system. Although he was influenced by the works of Locke and Boyle during his Oxford education, his oeuvre was written entirely within Galenic idiom, and his works often attempted to reinterpret Galenic notions in the context of new discoveries. *Medicina Gerocomica* is an exhaustive and encyclopaedic account of the Galenic aging body and its interaction with the outside world, explained with tireless precision and formality.

Structured around the identification of correct regimen for each corporeal temperament in old age, *Medicina Gerocomica* seems to advocate exactly what we might expect from a work of Galenic therapeutics. 'The best Physician for old Men', wrote Floyer in his opening pages, was one 'who knows the Medicines that will moisten and warm them'.[65] Ostensibly, *Medicina Gerocomica* is a work all about temperature. Floyer's aim was to describe how to access the properties of heat in the outside world, and how to bring the right amount of heat in to the aging body for maximum beneficial effect. In his efforts to do so he demonstrated a rather taxonomic impulse: Floyer set about listing and categorizing the heating and cooling properties of an endless number of external phenomena. Reading *Medicina Gerocomica*, one cannot help but get a sense of the perceived power of heat at large in the cosmos, and of Floyer's unremitting drive to classify where, when and how it might be accessed and administered.

The exact nature of the quality of 'heat' in Floyer's scheme is complex. The items listed under Floyer's 'hot' affective phenomena were not – at least to our modern eyes – 'hot' in a literal sense. They included some obvious entities like hot baths, hot fires, hot beds and hot 'cloaths'. Certain foods and drink could be denominated hot; 'hot Meats' being those that were 'acrid, bitter, salt, foetid' and 'aromatic'. Yet metaphysical experiences could have heating properties too: 'anger, Joy, Revenge, many Cares, much Study' and 'constant *Vigilae*', were categorized as having heating properties and considered detrimental for most aging bodies.[66] What connects these seemingly disparate affective phenomena in Floyer's scheme – foods, habits, emotions, clothes – is their ability to produce a direct and quantifiable effect on vital processes.

It would be misplaced to interpret Floyer's apparent focus on temperature too literally or rigidly. As Barbara Duden reminds us, the four grand qualities of hot, cold, wet and dry 'comprised something other than tangible degrees of moistness or temperature'.[67] Floyer's hot therapies did more than just 'heat' the body in the strictest sense of the word. The heat inherent in Floyer's list of chosen medicines and therapies both compliments and is compatible with the vital 'heat' inside the body: the essence of life itself. Like Cheyne's example of light and diluting foodstuffs, the heat in the macrocosm and heat in the microcosm are considered of a piece. However, Floyer's 'heat' has another property altogether, for its significance lies not only in the sensory register, but also in the temporal one. References to heat in *Medicina Gerocomica* are habitually qualified by Floyer's noting its effect on the pace or speed of physiological functioning, particularly that of the circulation and pulse. Heat, in other words, can literally speed up or slow down bodily function. As Floyer put it: 'All things' that 'accelerate the Pulse ... hasten old Age'.[68]

In practical terms then, the regulation of the aging body depended on knowing how, as Floyer put it, 'Non Naturals alter the Pulse'. As he went on to explain, 'hot Air ... stimulates the Heart to a greater and quick Circulation', whereas cold made the 'Pulse more rare, small, slow'.[69] Autumn and winter were the seasons 'most injurious to old Men', specifically because it was then that 'the Circulation and Pulses are most stopt'.[70] The 'hot' and 'cold' properties of the Non-naturals are, therefore, something of a shorthand for denominating the power to alter the functioning of body: to speed it up when it is sluggish and decaying, or slow it down when it is over-taxed in order to preserve the length of life. Floyer's concept of heat is emphatically not just the quality of being hot, as can be touched, tasted or felt; it is a *dynamic* force. It bespeaks vitality, energy: life itself. It is not so much a 'quality' or property but an agent, invested with the ability to affect the body's mechanism, to quicken the circulation, accelerate or retard the pulse, burn life quickly or slowly, compose and restore or disorder and expend.

Unregulated, the power of heat had the potential to wreak havoc on the body, and the aging body in particular. Such was Floyer's belief, and it was exactly this imagined danger that prompted him to champion the cause for which he was best known: the promotion of cold-water bathing. *The Ancient Psychrolousia Revived, or, An Essay to Prove Cold Bathing both Safe and Useful* (1702), reached six editions, and was the most published of his works. In addition to endorsing the practice in print, he established his own charitable cause, encouraging worthy and obliging men of Litchfield to contribute to the construction of cold public baths. Floyer developed a growing consternation about the body-heating, circulation-speeding and aging properties inherent within a host of lately fashionable practices and consumables. With the 'Increase and Interest of Foreign Trade in the last Century', there had been an influx of 'hot' stimulants such as 'Tobacco, Tea, Coffee, Wine, and Brandy-Spirits, and Spices'.[71] As these commodities were part of 'Hot Regimen from the Hot Climates' they were 'unnatural to English Bodies' and occasioned an undesirable warming and speeding effect. In order to combat the detrimental effects of such, Floyer suggested 'Cold Bathing' might be an appropriate and 'useful Practice'. When already contending with the various heating properties offered by new stimulants in a mercantile society, the very last thing that aging bodies needed was another warming influence in the form of a hot bath. A 'Hot' bath had the real potential to 'hasten Old Age, and shorten Life'.[72]

Floyer described the dangerous sensitivity of an aging body at the mercy of a changing outside world. Yet by the same token he was able to write a compendious work describing how to manage that body; describing in detail how it might respond to the Non-naturals, and how therefore it could be quite rationally controlled. Of course, Floyer's devotion to the Galenic scheme was not representative of the wider medical establishment, but his work does provide a sense of why these schemes might be so hypnotic and enduring in eighteenth-century minds, particularly when making sense of the aging body.

Conclusion

Put together, the various interpretative schemes discussed in this chapter provide a conceptual matrix for making sense of the aging body in eighteenth-century England. Yet these schemes were not the only frames of reference on offer at this point in time. Discussed in the following chapter are the new body models that were to supersede the old scheme to which Floyer was so attached. Still, in attempting to cover a number of different interpretative angles, I hope to have shown that the aging body in eighteenth-century England was something that could be understood on many levels: social, cosmological, spiritual and medical.

Aging was not a secular issue in eighteenth-century England. The weight of the Christian tradition continued to inform at a fundamental level ideas about the aging body: ideas about the historical specificity of the human body and human life, ideas connecting moral probity and physical decay, and ideas about the inherent virtue of moderation and abstention. Mixing doctrines from astrology, numerology, medicine and the life cycle, the notion of climacteric years served to present aging as a thing mysterious, superhuman and cosmological. In eighteenth-century England, many of the forces of aging were seen to come from the outside world. Within the descriptions examined here, the external world is accorded an extraordinary significance: an assumed ability to permeate the skin and produce a direct affect upon physiological function. 'The Body is consumed by external as well as internal Causes', explained Floyer, investing that statement – one imagines – with a degree of literalness that we will struggle to appreciate.[73]

Those who have researched the medical culture of eighteenth-century England have remarked upon the conservatism inherent in medical advice, and in particular the way in which it remained grounded within the parameters of the six Non-naturals. Despite both the burgeoning culture of health, the expansion of print and significant – paradigmatic – shifts in the theory of medicine, the content of many publications differed little from the teachings of the Ancients. Roy Porter saw this as amounting to a divide between theory and practice:

> Eighteenth century mechanistic approaches, with their vision of a body governed by universal laws of matter in motion, produced new physiological and pathological concepts. Yet, as so often in medicine, treatments changed less than the theories rationalising them.[74]

While there may have been some inherent conservatism in medical publications, the persistence of the old ways may actually be something to do with the way aging itself was understood. When medical texts addressed themselves to aging and longevity, the continued centrality of the Non-naturals is hardly surprising given that the body was certainly not yet seen to 'age' internally or biologically. As we will see in the following chapter, even the physiologists who coined the new mechanistic visions found it impossible to write about an aging process without imagining the contingent effects of various external Non-natural factors upon the body. This not only assured the endurance of a Galenic system of therapeutics in a medical culture otherwise attuned to material mechanism, but also reflects the way in which aging in particular continued to be perceived as an external as well as an internal phenomenon.

It does seem entirely intuitive that biological processes beneath the skin are not entirely autonomous or self-regulating. Even with our biologically skewed gazes in the twenty-first century, we are happy to acknowledge that external matter has a bearing on aging bodies. But in the case of the writings examined here, it is emphatically not the case that external forces *may* have an indirect, knock-on effect in the way that we hope various health measures may alleviate our aging problems today. External factors did not occupy a less significant place in the real causes of physiological aging. We must remember that environment and conditions of life continued to be seen as determining general levels of health in populations: this did not change until the 'bacteriological revolution' in the later nineteenth century.[75] Despite paradigm shifts in medical circles, the eighteenth-century body continued to occupy a deep significance beyond the reach of medicine: a significance that was cosmological, historical, biblical. It remained a multi-dimensional object with import way beyond its own materiality.

3 THE NEW SCIENCE: AGING AND AGENCY

Introduction

Thanks to a unique combination of enabling factors, eighteenth-century English medical writers could champion agency over aging bodies in new and exciting proportions. Managing and controlling the aging body seemed more possible and more tangible than it had ever before, and perhaps more so than it has seemed since. At base, much of this can be explained by the factors considered in previous chapters: the aging of the body was still conceived to have its loci in the outside world, and human lifespan was not yet considered universal or fixed. With such an epistemological framework in place it seems inevitable that aging might be considered an inherently manageable phenomenon. Yet as well as playing host to these already flexible epistemological underpinnings, the eighteenth century also saw the advent of some new ideas that made management of the aging body all the more feasible. New physiological paradigms and psychoperceptual schemes could be called upon to explain and endorse agency over the aging body in more stimulating and 'scientific' ways. Thanks furthermore to a burgeoning print culture in which medical texts could thrive and a cultural moment attuned to celebrating the performative aspects of bodiliness, agency over the aging body became a distinctive aspect of discourse. This was a historical moment at which agency over aging was fundamentally unproblematic, practically explicable and culturally apt.

Having taken a broad and multi-faceted approach in the previous chapter, this chapter focuses on practical, physiological interpretations of the aging body provided by the medical establishment. In addition to the established humoral scheme, there was a new and distinctly more 'scientific' vision that was breaking onto the scene at the dawn of the period under discussion here. In Western Europe, in the first half of the eighteenth century, two important medical men and latterday physiologists were to provide new models of bodily function that reconfigured the whole notion of life and its operations between cradle and grave. Within the new systems – the 'mechanistic' body and the 'sensible' body that it spawned – the human body could be reduced to a system of mechanical cause and effect.

The first part of this chapter is devoted to a close reading of the key texts that described the 'new' body to Western Europe – the works of the Dutch physiologist Herman Boerhaave (1669–1738) and his Swiss pupil Albrecht von Haller (1708– 77). In theory, these systems offered profound revisions for understanding the aging process. However, the advent of new physiological paradigms did not automatically dispel the more fundamental ideas about aging discussed in the previous chapter: these physiologists remained happy to locate the causes of aging in the outside world and the contingencies of human experience. The second half of the chapter demonstrates the practical repercussions of these new paradigms in the medical culture of eighteenth-century England. Boerhaave's ideas introduced some novel and useful ways of explaining what happened beneath the skin of an aging body, and it was via some of their new ideas, rules, laws, expressions and metaphors that writers of eighteenth-century English medical advice endorsed agency over the aging process. As a result of the new paradigmatic visions of body function, writers were able to imagine a newly accessible aging process. They were able to describe how it would respond in certain and newly quantifiable ways, and most importantly, how it could be subjected to rational self-control.

To date, there has been no specific study examining the impact of new physiological paradigms on advice about the management of the aging body. Within the history of medicine, a number of works have extrapolated and explained the workings of new body models, and others have demonstrated how these theories were presented to reading publics through the mechanism of print. There is a considerable body of literature that has considered how new philosophical and physiological paradigms informed eighteenth-century moral philosophy, and an ever-increasing number of studies examining how such theories gave birth to a 'cult' of sensibility, reflected especially in the novels and conduct literature of the period.[1] Aside from these studies of the sensible body, historical research on eighteenth-century medical advice as a genre has tended to emphasize its relative conservatism in structure, content and tone, and (as we saw at the end of the previous chapter) its continued adherence to prescription via the Non-naturals.

However, one project that combines a focus on the mechanistic paradigm with the history of old age is that by Daniel Schafer. Schafer's study focuses on the perceived status of old age in European medical texts, considering constructions of both old age and diseased bodies across the early modern period.[2] He argues that the advent of the mechanistic body model was a central component in cementing the notion that old age was pathological. This, he believes, can be explained by the fact that mechanism brought about a new concept of disease itself. In strictly mechanistic terms, all change from normality was considered dysfunctional and pathological, and within this schema, the final part of life could be considered just that. Conceding that it had been possible to think of old age as a disease since the ancients, Schafer claims that it was after 1650 in particular that there was a marked tendency to medicalize and pathologize old age. However, he also draws attention to a surprising fact: there were no 'practical consequences' of this tendency. That is, no disciplines of gerontology or geriatric pathology were actually developed to investigate and medicate this so-called disease. This chapter takes a rather different approach, focusing not on the way in which old age was presented in eighteenth-century texts, but on the ways in which eighteenth-century writers wrote about *managing* the aging body.

A New Paradigm: Boerhaave and Haller Formulate the Aging Machine

Historians of science, medicine and philosophy are well aware that by the end of the seventeenth century, developments in medicine and intellectual thought known collectively as the 'scientific revolution' had radically challenged accepted modes of interpreting the cosmological and terrestrial order. This 'Newtonising' of knowledge, and 'deontologizing of the world of matter' enabled alternative visions of the body, and alternative medical practices.[3] In 1628, William Harvey published his anti-Galenic conclusion that the blood continually circulated around the body, driven by a heart that functioned as a pump. The mid-seventeenth-century saw the emergence of Descartes's radical theory that the living body worked mechanically, just 'a watch of any other AUTOMA' and was not kept alive and in motion by any activity of the soul.[4] In England, in the 1660s, the anatomist Thomas Willis identified the soul with the brain and argued that the nerves alone were held responsible for sensory impressions, and consequently for knowledge. John Locke, his student, systemized Willis's sensational psychology into a philosophical theory in his *Essay Concerning Human Understanding* (1690). Throughout the eighteenth century, the importance accorded to 'nerves, spirits and fibres' was to inform moral philosophy, and as G. J. Barker-Benfield has demonstrated, this sparked a wider 'culture of sensibility'.[5]

As a broad consequence of these and other developments, medical theory was losing its links with classical teaching: the role of the humours was no longer called upon to explain disease and physiological dysfunction. Instead, the Cartesian metaphor of mechanical causation allowed the body to be viewed as a reactive machine. Within the new science, it was Herman Boerhaave and his pupil Albrecht von Haller who in the 1710s and 1740s wrote the seminal texts for the new paradigm. These visions – those that we have come to recognize as the mechanistic body and the sensible body – were to prove dominant in explaining life's functions in Western Europe from the early eighteenth century onwards.

Under the direction of Boerhaave, the leading medical school of Leiden was to become the centre of 'physiology', a new term supposedly coined by Boerhaave himself.[6] Boerhaave also authored the standard 'textbook' for the new science, his *Institutiones Medicae* (1715). English translations appeared immediately, followed by numerous further editions and formats throughout the century. At the heart of this new science was Boerhaave's reformulation of body function: by formatting Cartesian mechanism into medical idiom, Boerhaave created a body model known as 'hydraulic mechanism'. According to him, life was a question of bodily structures and pressures, and health depended on the unobstructed motion of essential fluids. Unlike the old humoral body, it did not experience elemental fluctuations, but worked mechanically. Every last movement and any functional process were isolatable and detectable. 'The Human Body', he wrote in his opening section, 'Of Physiology', in the *Institutiones Medicae*,

> is compos'd as Anatomical Enquiries teach us, of Solids and Fluids; The Solids are, either Vessels that contain the Fluids, or Instruments so formed, configurated and connected, that certain determinate Motions may be perform'd or exercis'd from this single Fabrick, if any moving Cause concur. For there we find Supporters, Pillars, Clothing or Covering, Partitions, Rollers, Wedges, Leavers, Pullies, Cords, Presses, Bellows, Sieves, Strainers, Canals and Receptacles. The faculty of exercising these Motions is call'd a Function, which is agreeable to the Laws of Mechanism, by which only it can be explain'd.[7]

As this section will demonstrate, the vision of body function conceived by Boerhaave and later modified by Haller allowed the first recognizably 'scientific' description of physical aging. It was via the works of these leading European medical men that the body's changes between birth and death were demystified, explained and internalized. Although neither addressed the subject of aging directly, a close reading of their ideas about body function reveals how – at a theoretical level – this new paradigm was enormously significant for the very concept of aging itself. In fact, I argue that Boerhaave and Haller provided a nascent vision of aging as a biological process; in some ways their ideas were recognizably modern. Henceforth, I will refer to my interpretation of their ideas about the aging body as the formulation of an 'aging machine'.

The aging machine did not decline on account of its depletion of natural heat. Boerhaave offered a new explanation for why aging occurred. At a basic level, aging was now explicable in terms of the circulation and motion of fluids in the body. According to Boerhaave, the journey through life was a continual metamorphosis from fluid to solid, regulated by internal processes of circulation and motion. Physical decline came about as a result of an impaired circulation, which in turn was exacerbated by insufficient nourishment from circulating juices. The body was still reckoned to become drier and harder, but these factors were now seen as the mere manifestations of aging rather than the physical cause. The failure of the circulation starved the body of requisite nourishment, and this produced dryness and hardness both internally and externally. Hence Boerhaave provided a more tangible and material interpretation for what had previously been accounted for by the rather ethereal, enigmatic concept of declining 'vital heat'. Essentially, Boerhaave described a nexus of cause and effect within the body, a mutually reinforcing trajectory that necessitated and internalized material decline and decay. In theory then, aging could now be seen as a far more internal, regulated phenomenon.

Perhaps the most memorable aspect of Boerhaave's Cartesian-inspired formula was the fact that the body was now to be imagined and described as a machine. Aging was equated with a machine's 'wearing out'. The gradual failure of the circulatory principle and the consequent restriction of the nourishing juices was likened to a machine becoming gradually less effective, rickety and eventually redundant. Like any piece of mechanical equipment, the body would wear down with repeated daily use. And because the body was being used all the time, it wore away incrementally and predictably as it moved, lived and breathed; a result of the daily 'actions of Life', as Boerhaave put it.[8] Boerhaave imagined a body that, just by nature of being alive, had to endure a great deal of wear and tear. He mused on the 'violent and perpetual Motions our soft tender Machines sustain during the Space of so many Years', and thought it only logical that these continual abrasive effects would eventually destroy it.[9] Boerhaave's equation of the body with a machine was entirely literal: during life, parts of the machine might break off; others could be rubbed away or ground down. For as he was at pains to emphasize, the fact that motions were '*continually* and violently performed in Vessels of such a *tender* Fabric',

> must necessarily occasion the smallest Parts to be broke or rubbed off from the solid Fibres by the continual Impulse of the Humours and Actions of the Muscles ... in the mean time the Fluids [are] continually lessened, or ground small by Attrition ... from hence the living Machine of the Animal *soon* destroys itself from the very Condition of its Frame.[10]

Over the course of a normal life, the physical condition of the body would change immeasurably: it started out soft tender pliant and became brittle, hard and stiff. 'A Thorough sound Body', wrote Boerhaave, 'by Actions that are inseparable from a healthful Condition of Life, by degrees is so chang'd'. In later life, he explained, 'the smallest Fibres become rigid or stiff ... the finest Vessels grow into concreted Fibres', and 'the larger Vessels harden and close'.[11] Incremental hardening of the body's tissues meant it was increasingly difficult for the fluids to circulate. Eventually, he explained, all the tissues and fibres were 'drawn together, growing each to the other, from whence comes Dryness, want of Motion, and a Decay of Age'.[12] Ultimately, the body became so hard and inelastic that it impeded its own function, providing 'too great Resistance' for the Heart to manage.[13] Herein was what Boerhaave described as the 'kind of Death which follows from mere old Age'.[14] By internalizing the process of aging, and making it attendant on the most fundamental 'actions of life', Boerhaave rendered aging entirely inevitable.

What was novel about Boerhaave's formulation was the idea that the body destroyed itself by the nature of its own function. 'The living Machine of the Animal *soon* destroys itself from the very Condition of its Frame', he explained.[15] Cause and effect were now visible beneath the skin; in fact they were written into the material structure of the body itself. Decay was intrinsic to the corporeal mass. So, in mechanistic terms, aging was inseparable from the concept of life. It was not so much that bodies 'aged', or began to age at some point, but rather that existence from birth to death was part of the same mutually reinforcing mechanical trajectory. To use an anachronistic expression, Boerhaave essentially recognized that aging was – in the words of contemporary gerontologists – a 'lifelong process', for the living machine was constantly, gradually destroying itself from the moment of its inception.[16] 'The Body naturally destroys itself from its own Nature', Boerhaave noted, 'and the Animal no sooner begins to live, than to approach towards Death, which is the Consequence of Life'.[17] Yet despite articulating one of the key tenets of modern social gerontology long *avant la lettre* Boerhaave did not isolate the concept of an aging 'process' or furnish it with its own terms.

Around mid-century, Boerhaave's theory was being complemented by visions of bodies imbued with more animate, vital properties.[18] Emphasis was moving from the vascular to the nervous system as the locus of vitality, and significance was placed upon the identifiable qualities of irritability, sensibility and excitability. 'Sensibility' denoted the operation of the nervous system; the material basis for consciousness as systematized in the psycho perceptual schemes of Newton and Locke. It was Boerhaave's student, the Swiss physiologist, and professor of anatomy, surgery and medicine at Gottingen and later Bern, Albrecht von Haller who was responsible for producing the next generation of academic textbooks to formulate these modifications. At Leiden, Haller made sensibility into a physiological property open to investigation and experiment. He described 'neural man', a phrase that connoted the innate animation of the nerves (separate from the mind's rational capacities), which stirred the body to life and quickened the interaction of mind and body. It is Haller's oeuvre that has traditionally been credited with describing the 'vitalist' model of the body, and his textbooks developed the hydraulic body into a more sensitive machine. Haller's reputation was international, and nowhere was he more recognized than in England, where he became a fellow of the Royal Society in 1743 and was ennobled by George II in 1749. His key text, *First Lines of Physiology* was available in English translation by 1754, and a further seven English language translations followed. Similarly, the extended *Elementa Physiologiae Corporis Humani* (1757–66) remained in print until the end of the century.

Mechanism and vitalism were not opposed or incompatible paradigms, but essentially variations on a theme. Both worked mechanically, but the sensible body placed more emphasis on the inherent responsiveness of tissues imbued with nerves. As Andrew Wear points out, despite the emphatic shift from the vascular to nervous systems, throughout the eighteenth century 'leading medical theorists agreed that elucidation of the body depended upon "systematic investigation of fibres and vessels"'.[19] Indeed, outside faculty medicine and academic physiology, theoretical distinctions often disappeared. As John Mullan has noted in *Sentiment and Sociability* (1988), within eighteenth-century conduct books and novels, 'there is scarcely a separation between vocabularies of "feeling" and "passion", on the one hand, and of anatomically considered mechanism, on the other'.[20]

The shifted emphasis from vascular to nervous body structure did not, in any essential way, influence how Haller dealt with the 'aging' of the body. In *First Lines of Physiology* (1786), Haller offered an expanded analysis of the changes the body underwent through the life course based essentially on Boerhaave's functional-mechanical description. Faithful student of Boerhaave that he was, Haller addressed the phenomenon of aging under a final chapter entitled 'Nutrition, Growth, Life and Death'.[21] Life was continued growth; growth eventually brought about death, and the intermitting periods involved growing and decaying: it was all of a piece. Aging was therefore a lifelong process. As Haller explained, 'we feel the beginnings of decay even in youth itself'.[22]

Like that of his teacher, Haller's core conception of aging was of a body ground down by the wear and tear brought about by its own movements and functions. 'The cause of the destruction' of the body was to be located in the 'perpetual extension and retraction' of its moving parts.[23] This, Haller was keen to point out, happened 'at every pulse of the heart ... an hundred thousand times every day'. There was, of course, no way to escape the body's continual frictions; it was utterly inevitable, and best accepted. 'We are all perpetually consuming', Haller wrote blithely, 'all parts of our body are the sooner worn away'.[24] Haller was particularly prone to endorsing the body-machine equation, and he likened the friction of body's parts to the chafing of metal cogs and components.[25] He also pointed out that wear and tear on the aging machine was not uniform, rather 'those parts grow stiff soonest which are most exercised by motion', he explained, and noted that much the same could be said for 'any mechanic' and the tools 'which he chiefly makes use of in his business'.[26] Haller's lively mechanical metaphors were to make more visually persuasive the concept of real wear and tear that was now both the metaphorical – and literal – explanation for physical aging. Not surprisingly, these discernible metaphors and allusions translated well into English medical advice.

The Theoretical Legacy of Mechanism for the Aging Body

At a philosophical and ideological level, the mechanistic body threatened to reconfigure the entire concept of aging. Unlike its humoral predecessor, the aging machine functioned on its own terms rather than at some mysterious cosmological level. Material mechanism gave the body its own existential autonomy. The 'aging' of the body was now visible and explicable, for mechanism located a nexus of cause and effect *within* the body, or as Boerhaave had put it, 'the Body naturally destroys itself from its own Nature'.[27] Theoretically, in this mechanical view, there was no room for imagining abstract natural or cosmological forces determining internal processes: the body simply wore itself out. Furthermore, Boerhaave and Haller gave explicit recognition to the fact that they considered aging to be a *process*, a lifelong process.[28] Haller had noted that 'we feel the beginnings of decay even in youth itself'.[29] In short, mechanism seems to have brought about the possibility of describing an aging process in a truly modern sense: recognition that aging was a discrete, steady and internally regulated biological process that happened between cradle and grave.

However, neither Boerhaave nor Haller developed an independent term or idea to convey an idea of 'aging' in its own right. Neither isolated the subject for independent consideration. Both men continued to frame their researches in the established interpretative frameworks of lifecycle and cosmos. Boerhaave still talked about life in ages, stages and 'Seasons'. At the outset of his work he framed his heuristic parameters thus:

> Which be the difference of Structure of the Solid Parts in the different Ages of Life? Why man grows, continues for some Years of the same height; and afterwards in old Age grows short again, and less? Why he is sometimes of a loose texture, sometimes of a strong and stiff one? Why he is sometimes Moist and full, at other times Dry? ... What Distempers are most common to each particular Age? What Diet, what sort of Life, what Medicines are the most adapted to the several Seasons of Life?[30]

Even though his formulations seemed to refute the legitimacy of a stagistical model of life, it seems it was just inconceivable for him to think outside the concept of the life cycle as a mental ordering strategy.

Boerhaave and Haller emphatically did not envisage human lifespan as a universal biological principle. In their writings, lifespan was not so much a chronological trajectory, but a functional one. Life ended not at a certain biologically ordained point or window (for example, sixty or ninety years), but when the machine wore out. The amount of time this might take was considered entirely flexible. Boerhaave located the impediments to longevity at a *physical* rather than *fundamental* level. 'If a Person could prevent the smallest Vessels from concreting into Fibres', he reasoned, 'he might render Life perpetual'.[31] Although he quickly stated that this was something that (at his present time) 'no

Mortal can effect', the theoretical possibility remained.[32] Aging machines had no particular biologically determined shelf life. Human life was still, in the minds of these scientists, a historically specific and contingent phenomenon; and an inherently flexible one too.

Furthermore, Boerhaave and Haller continued to discuss aging – or in their terms, the 'decay' of the body – as heavily determined by the forces of nature. Although they acknowledged that a body would wear out as a result of its internal mechanisms, the exact pace at which it wore out, and the amount of damage incurred was still understood to be highly dependent on the world outside. When Haller explained that it was the 'actions of life' that exhausted the body, this was not just 'life' beneath the skin, but life in its fullest, autobiographical sense: a human being's interaction with the outside world. Haller did not hesitate to look beyond the skin to isolate the determinants of physical aging. The coming of 'old age', as Haller termed it, was necessarily contingent and subjective:

> The hardness or rigidity of the whole body, the decrease of the muscular powers, and the weakening of the senses, constitute *old age*; which happens to mankind sometimes sooner, and sometimes later: sooner if they have been subjected to violent labour, or given themselves up to pleasure, or lived upon unwholesome diet: but more slowly if they have followed a moderate way of life, and used temperance in their diet, or if they have removed from a cold to a warm country.[33]

There was still no template for 'normal' body aging; aging machines were run by individual mechanics in very different situations and with very different effects. Despite wearing out in more scientific and subcutaneous ways, the aging machine still wore out at a subjective and contingent pace, and was still highly responsive to unpredictable forces in the world outside.

It is essential to remember that these new paradigms for physiological function were explanatory mechanisms that operated at a physical rather than a fundamental level. The arrival of mechanistic ideas about the aging body could complement rather than challenge some of the more foundational and indispensable tenets about aging examined in the previous chapter. Physiological theories are not necessarily capable of debunking ideas about the spiritual significance of the aging body; developments in the realm of science do not have to be attended by movements towards secularization. Physiological theories, however progressive, cannot be seen in isolation from the broad epistemological frameworks with which they were, after all, conceived. Likewise, progressive physiologists, however scientifically minded, were not exempt from thinking about the aging body in all its spiritual, cosmological, technicolour significance. Boerhaave still made reference to climacteric years, and talked about life in 'Seasons'. Both he and Haller still envisaged a body made up of the four elemental properties of the universe. Certainly, mechanism provided new ways to account for physical decline, but ultimately this great paradigm shift did not displace the great, broad, cosmological significance of the aging body.

Medical Advice Literature

The ideas discussed above belong to the exalted realms of European academic physiology. In the medical culture of eighteenth-century England, the impact of such ideas was necessarily limited. In the more popular and accessible material, these new scientific ideas did not translate uniformly or purely. Body models were not watertight or mutually exclusive, and often overlapped. In lay medical advice the body was often described as an assemblage of various body models. Sometimes it was described as a bucket of humours, hydraulic machine or bundle of sensitive nerves, but it was just as likely to be a body that had elements of all of these configurations. This is not to say that the new science did not make some impact on writings about the aging body; it did. But its impact was one of degree rather than kind. Mechanism did not bring about a new vision of aging, or a new system of advice for the aging body. Instead it enabled an extension of the imagined parameters for self-mastery. In eighteenth-century medical advice, the key idea that mechanism was called upon to express was one about agency over physical decay and the possibilities of psychosomatic self-control. Although the aging body had always been presented as requiring management and discipline in popular health and medical writings, it was via the new idiom that the relationship between aging and agency became more intimate.

Also, in the hands of writers with a democratic agenda, mechanistic ideas provided some of the core ideological foundations for describing an essentially manageable, interactive aging body. Although we should not be surprised to see those who authored medical advice advocating active engagement with the body, there is something more rudimentary present here than the demands of form. The role of the human agent in managing the aging process is not only implied in these texts but also positively, explicitly endorsed, rendered empirically defensible and even defined as necessary. Activity beneath the skin was denoted highly interactive; the vital processes that facilitated decay were considered responsive and pliable. In the works of medical advice we find not only the sentiments to endorse management of the body, but the practical guidelines through which it could be achieved: the instructions to enable real physical change beneath the skin.

Although regimen continued to be formalized under the rubric of the six Non-naturals, it was now possible to write about a scientifically fathomable machine that would respond to them in formulaic and tangible ways. Indeed, the Non-naturals themselves could be presented as the very laws and rules with which 'any mechanic' could operate and discipline their own aging machine. Edward Strother, the physician who edited Boerhaave's works for the English market, opened his *Essay on Sickness and Health* by echoing Boerhaave's sentiment about the functional potential for immortality inherent in the human frame: 'If we had the Art of managing [the Non-naturals] mathematically, it were possible to prolong Life, to a great period'.[34] Strother's 1729 *Family Companion for Health*, claimed to offer 'rules' which would 'infallibly' procure 'long life' for his readers. Allusions to mechanical rules and laws pervade medical texts, as do sentiments about the body's user-friendliness. Writers of eighteenth-century medical advice often presented themselves as authoring instruction manuals for the mechanical operation of the aging machine.

These sentiments found expression in mechanical idiom. Writers explained that the aging of the body was a process of 'wearing out', a phrase lifted directly from the works of Boerhaave and Haller. Whether or not writers referenced these eminent physiologists explicitly, this was the favoured shorthand for describing the nature of physical decline. It was also an implicit means of determining that aging was a functional and subjective process. Writers focused on the fact that a body wore out functionally. Therefore, as it was possible to manage the 'use' to which the aging machine was put, it was entirely possible to manage the *rate* at which it aged, and consequently the length of life that could be lived. 'Wearing out' became an expression of agency and empowerment. Advice often took the form of suggesting how wear and tear upon the body might be minimized, or even removed. The key to management of the aging machine was to minimize use, and if that was impossible, then it was necessary to keep the machine extremely well oiled.

For Cheyne, the body was a sensible, pliable machine, responsive to the soul and vulnerable to the outside world. If its use was gentle and moderate, then its process of wearing out would be likewise. Cheyne's discussion of the aging body was characterized by a desire to expose its internal mechanics in some detail, thereby demonstrating the inherent pliability of vital processes to carefully chosen management strategies. The first step to rational body management, he explained, was to get acquainted with the mechanics of physical decay. Hence Cheyne presented an extended description of physical decline based on Boerhaave's account in the *Institutiones Medicae*. He set about detailing how the blood begins to thicken, to move around sluggishly, to be restricted and unable to complete efficient circulatory rounds: 'The Blood and Juices ... begin to *cool*, to *thicken*, to become *vapid*, and to be *obstructed* in the *Capillaries* and *Lymphatics*'.[35] As 'the *Circulation* [is] gradually reduced into a narrowe Compass', the very fabric of the body becomes more solid, resistant and impenetrable, harder in its very essence. 'Natural *Death* by reason of Age only', he explained, was effected by cooling and 'thickening [of] the Blood, which gradually lessens the Extent of, and finally stops, the *Circulation*'.[36]

Cheyne's impetus in opening up the aging body was to enable his readers to appreciate how entirely flexible and malleable these internal processes were.

In his vision, the fact of these vital processes being essential and subcutaneous did not render them involuntary. Inherent in the way in which he described the circulatory principle and the hardening of the body was an assumption that they were responsive to human intervention. Indeed, he wrote about their function and their manipulation in the same breath. It was simple: if the circulatory principle was reduced on account of circulating fluids becoming thicker and slower, then one should just keep those juices as thin and fluid as possible. Cheyne knew that there were things that could work on the body's fluids to keep them supple and pliant. Once these could be applied – rather like the action of oiling a machine – its vital processes would respond and keep it working for longer. It was no more complex than eating a 'meager and diluting Diet'. [37] A thin diet allowed the 'Blood and Juices' to be kept within a 'due State of Thinness and Fluidity', enabling the 'Rounds and Circulations' to be made with the 'fewest Rubs and least Resistance'. Knowing how to keep the aging machine well oiled and nicely fluid was to minimize the fatal wear and tear – or 'Rubs' and 'Resistance' as Cheyne put it. This was, in short, the 'Grand Secret and Sole Mean of Long Life'.[38] The longevity of the machine was within the hands of the mechanic; all that was required was a supply of the right fluids.

The ideology of 'wearing out' had a particularly diachronic emphasis; it was especially instructive for the management of aging. As Cheyne explained, care of the body in the here-and-now had an inevitably long-term corollary. Wisdom, prudence and correct regimen could ensure 'a lively rational *Head* under *Silver Hairs*, and a vigorous active *Heart* to animate even a feeble decaying *Trunk*'.[39] As he told his readers, 'the *Faculties* and their *Senses* ... may, by a wise and prudent *Oeconomy*, be supported to the very last Stage of Life'.[40] Although Cheyne was as wedded to pious abstention and the Non-naturals as any eighteenth-century health writer, his ideology and philosophy were informed by a new and excited sense of a body fathomable and knowable. No body mechanism was beyond the reach of human intervention. Ultimately, when it came to preserving health and achieving longevity, 'The Means', he wrote, 'are mostly in our own Power'.[41]

The physician-actor John Hill (who was in fact a correspondent of Haller's) did much to champion the great potential for human agency over a body that could now be understood as a reactive, fathomable mechanism. It was through a close acquaintance with Haller's physiology that Hill was able to posit his wholehearted belief in agency and couch this belief in scientific fact. In his two health and longevity guides written in the 1750s and 1760s, Hill presented his readers with a vision of an aging body that – with the right management – could be brought entirely under rational control. Hill, like Cheyne, offered his readers a synopsis of the subcutaneous mechanisms that accounted for symptomatic aging and natural death – a simplified version of Haller's scheme. 'We live by perfect circulation; we decline as it becomes impaired; and when it stops we die', he summarized.[42] However, it was also important for him to explain at rather greater length what this principle involved, for the secret of mastery was to be found in a sophisticated and detailed awareness of the aging machine:

> In the prime of life the larger arteries contract and expand strongly, and freely: their contraction forces the blood forward, with a strength that carries it through the most distant and small vessels in the extreme parts; and their expansion afterwards gives free room to the heart, the seat and source of life, to throw into them the blood it has received from the veins, in consequence of their first motion. While this is well performed we live, and are in health: but age brings on a hardness in the larger vessles, and that impedes their motion. The force being weakened which drove the blood forward, it stops in many of the smaller vessels at the extremities; and old mens hands, and feet from hence grow lean, and cold; for warmth and nourishment are its gift: at last these larger vessels grow mere bone; they can contract, they can dilate no more; the heart unable to force into them the blood it has received from the veins, ceases to beat; and life ceases with it. This is the death of age, without disease: thus old men die merely by being old.[43]

'Thus in age we perish by degrees', Hill explained, 'and lose in every step some strength of sense and faculties'.[44] As this extract demonstrates, Hill appears to have a clear and conscious sense that aging is a process, and a natural and inevitable one at that. 'Death has a thousand doors to rush upon us; but this by which he makes his slow and regular advance is always open', he confirmed.[45] Like Cheyne, Hill interpreted these doctrines in a very positive way. His purpose in providing such a description for his readers was, by his own admission, pedagogical: 'when the cause is plain before us, we know at least which way to direct our course in trying to retard it'.[46] Knowledge was the way to successful management. Hill offered his readers something of an explanatory mission statement in the preface to his *Virtues of Sage in Lengthening Life*:

> If we would rationally attempt to lengthen Life, we must attend first to the causes of its decay. The human frame, made for a limited time, contains within itself the means of its destruction; the body wears away by use, nor can we prevent it: but by attending to the cause of this decline, we may put back the evil hour, and make its progress easier.[47]

Here, Hill makes explicit reference to Boerhaave's nexus of cause and effect within the body. Knowing that the human body contained 'within itself the means of its destruction', and knowing that it 'wears away by use' were the platforms upon which a programme of successful management could be based. Once rendered transparent, the 'rational' means for preventing its decline can be isolated. After all, the 'cause' of decline, as Hill explained, was no more than 'use' – something that it was entirely possible to control. By consequence, the pace or 'progress' of aging was entirely actionable. 'The management of life', Hill stated, 'is always in our power: a few plain rules for it, compleat the purpose of this little treatise.'[48] For Hill, the new body was a site of willed performance and self-control. It is perhaps no surprise that Hill wrote a discourse on the art of acting in which he explained – via a physiological system of cause and effect – how bodies could be trained to change on demand.[49] Based on his understanding of Haller's physiology, Hill described how the actor could morph into new physiological configurations for aesthetic effect. Discernible excitement about the limits of agency over mechanical bodies – whether on the stage or in life – characterized his work.

Whereas Boerhaave and Haller had concentrated on the *internal* process of wear and tear, medical advice writers tended to give the ideology of 'wearing out' a more *external* aspect. Wear and tear was often equated with the effects of the Non-naturals on the body. In the proffered interpretations, wear and tear was presumed to come from (or at least be regulated by) contingency, choice and the outside world. The central and empowering logic behind Buchan's *Domestic Medicine* of 1769 was the certainty that bodies were simply 'worn out' over the life course. They could be worn out sooner or later, depending on the particular uses to which they were put. Use was the all-important factor, and could be mediated by personal choice. Buchan explained that certain actions that required more use, effort or 'force', wore out the body at a faster pace and brought the body closer to death. Hence those who laboured in 'employments which necessarily require a great exertion of strength, as blacksmiths, carpenters, &c', were heading for a speedy decline on account of the 'violent' strain to which they subjected their bodies. He also thought that 'those who bear heavy burdens' were 'obliged to draw in the air with much greater force, and so to keep their lungs distended with more violence', with the result that the body would 'soon be worn out, and a premature old age brought on'.[50]

It was not only physical actions that destroyed the aging machine. In his section on 'Aliment', Buchan explained how the properties inherent in food and drink contained the potential to strain or exert the body, speeding up the pace at which vital reserves were expended, and hence accelerating the aging process. The heating influence of 'Fermented liquors' would encourage the blood to race around the body in a feverish fashion, rather in the same way that Floyer had feared might happen in a hot bath. 'They keep up a constant fever, which exhausts the spirits, heats and inflames the blood, and disposes the body to numberless diseases', he explained. 'Men who never take strong liquors ... live much longer than those who use them daily.' The acceleration and exhaustion they occasioned in the body wore out or 'wasted' the 'powers of life', and 'occasion[ed] premature old age'.[51]

Although the images of grinding down and wearing out had a very physical quality about them, a remarkable amount of attention was given to the mind and its ability to occasion wear and tear. Mental processes were considered just as abrasive for the aging machine, particularly when they strained over-delicate nerves. Cheyne described how excessive, intense thinking had the effect of 'wearing out the Body, as the Sword does the Scabbard'.[52] Similarly, Buchan remarked that 'man is evidently not formed for continual thought more than for perpetual action', and 'would soon be worn out by the one as by the other'.[53] When the physician and 'mad doctor' John Monro refuted as a 'vulgar error' the belief that madmen were likely to achieve longevity on account of their resistance to changes in temperature, he suggested an alternative thesis based on mental exertion. A distinct lack of mental activity, he thought, would probably ensure a kind of physical preservation. It was not especially 'madmen' therefore who were 'long lived', rather longevity was 'the lot of those only whose mental faculties seem to be totally obliterated, and who shew little or no attention to any thing that passes'. Low-grade, low-tolling mental exertion 'joined to [a] regular manner in which to live, will carry a strong, healthy constitution to a great age' he confirmed.[54]

For those who were capable of rational thought, however, psychosomatic self-control could be an important way of managing the aging process and achieving long life. The ability to comprehend the body as a 'sensible' mechanism with particular responsiveness to 'feelings' rendered the aging machine especially susceptible to being worn out and ground down by its cerebral and emotional experiences. Central to the concept of sensibility was an awareness that the sensitivity of nerve structures varied considerably between individuals. The degree, nature and intensity of mental operations were considered entirely dependent upon the relative pliability or rigour of the individual's nerves and intellectual faculties. Those of weaker, more sensitive nerves felt more strongly the impressions made upon their senses. As a consequence, weak nerves would be sooner worn and torn, and sooner worn out.

It was George Cheyne who was responsible for familiarizing eighteenth-century readers with the idea that certain people might be more sensible than others. He imagined nothing less than a tripartite class system, outlining this nervous hierarchy in a chapter on 'The Passions' in his *Essay*.[55] Cheyne explained that the difference in people's 'constitutions' depended on the relative pliability and elasticity of their nerves, and the proneness of these 'Fibres' to sensation. In Cheyne's scheme, those of the first nervous 'class' were those of *'springy, lively, and elastic* Fibres'. These sorts were imaginative, vivacious artistic people given to sensual and aesthetic pleasures. As discourse on the theatre makes clear, the celebrated theatre manager and actor David Garrick was a particular example of a very sensible constitution in the opinion of many of his eulogists.[56] Such persons, Cheyne thought, had 'the *quickest Sensations*', because 'a weaker *Impulse*' was able to produce 'a stronger *Sensation*' in their more delicate structures. By contrast, those of *'rigid, stiff, and unyielding* Fibres', Cheyne explained, had '*less vivid Sensations*', simply because it required 'a greater Degree of *Force* to overcome a greater *Resistance*'. These were the sorts of people who thought slowly and carefully, and excelled intellectually. 'Lastly', as Cheyne noted,

> those whose *Organs of Sensation* are (if I may speak so) *un-elastick*, or intirely *callous, resty* for want of Exercise, or any way *obstructed* or naturally *ill-informed*, as they have scare any *Passions* at all, or any lively Sensations, and are incapable of lasting *Impressions*; so they enjoy the *firmest* Health, and are subject to the fewest *Diseases*: such are *Ideots, Peasants* and *Mechanicks*, and all those we call Indolent People.[57]

Whereas the old scheme of humoral temperaments had provided a way of conceptualizing the differences in aging between individuals, this alternative vision of 'constitutions' (one that was not, by any means, incompatible with residual ideas about relative quantities of heat and moisture), explained why some bodies were sooner worn out than others. As Cheyne explained, men of feeling were unlikely to be long-lived as their sensitive, delicate nerves offered less resistance against wear and tear. Rather, the 'Ideots, Peasants and Mechanicks' were the ones who would be most likely enjoy long life. Cheyne made quite explicit his belief that 'Men of *Imagination*' were unlikely to enjoy great longevity: it was, as he put it 'hardly possible'.[58]

For this reason, actors were not considered likely to be long-livers. In mechanistic idiom, acting was a profession that involved an extraordinary amount of wear and tear. Those who combined physical exertion with phenomenal feats of the imagination – transporting themselves into quite another character no less – put their delicate machines under tremendous strain. As Roger Pickering was at pains to point out in his *Reflections upon Theatrical Expression in Tragedy* (1755), proper 'acting' was a very taxing holistic bodily exercise. 'Theatrical expression', he wrote involved 'every Attitude of every member of the Human Fabrick', as well as 'several Workings of the MIND'.[59] Acting manuals universally supported the notion that acting was hard graft, and would undoubtedly deplete on the body. 'Of all the Employments in Life, I know none so arduous in every Respect as that of a *Player*',[60] wrote the anonymous correspondent to the *Gentleman's Magazine* in 1743. Indeed, replicating the 'Rise and Progress of the Passions, together with their Effects on the Organs of our Bodies' on the boards every night took its toll; for passionate experience on the stage, just as in real life, involved considerable wearing of the machine.[61] In his *Life of Samuel Johnson*, Boswell reported a Johnsonian anecdote to similar effect. When Dr Burney 'remarked that Mr. Garrick was beginning to look old', Johnson apparently returned, 'Why, Sir, you are not to wonder at that; no man's face has had more wear and tear.'[62]

At face value, we could argue that the idea of a nerve hierarchy placed more emphasis on biological determinants for longevity, as the qualities of nerves and fibres were inherent and permanent. Whereas a raw mechanistic body could react in particular and predictable ways, vitalism required more emphasis to be placed on innate configurations of the nervous system. Differences in the degree of nervous pliability from person to person accounted for differing degrees of sensibility. The vitalistic body could therefore be considered to have a more in-built, predestined way of functioning that could jeopardize the degree to which it might be brought under conscious control. Yet this did not dampen the sense that aging was a malleable process, in fact, quite the opposite. Sensibility endorsed the more fundamental mechanistic assumption that action – or sensation – involved physical wear and tear, and so by protecting delicate nerves from straining experience, life could be prolonged. Although sensibility was an inherent disposition, the actual factors that twanged on delicate nerves came from the outside world. (Ultimately, sensibility was experience of the world outside via the sensory system.) The essential equation between 'use' and longevity was untouched, indeed endorsed. Contingency and choice was still just as important when it came to understanding the factors that aged the sensible body. However, it was through the ideology and idiom of the sensible body that psychosomatic therapies became an important part of managing and exercising agency over the aging body. Managing passions and sensations, keeping the right company, or simply thinking the right thoughts became an important part of eighteenth century ideas about aging, and this we will see in more detail in the following chapter.

Via these new languages of material mechanism and its attendant rhetoric of sensibility, life itself could be seen as distinctly abrasive for the aging machine. Flights of the imagination might be just as harmful as physical exertion for a body that wore away with even the slightest action or motion; and it followed that those who subjected their bodies to the greatest physical or emotional strain were hardly likely to achieve longevity. Yet the vulnerability of the new body – particularly the passionate, sensitive body – was also the quality that made it peculiarly responsive to management.

Conclusion

This chapter has considered the impact of new physiological paradigms on eighteenth-century ideas about the aging body, and in particular their impact upon the perceived relationship between aging and agency. In considering both the theoretical and the practical legacy of mechanism, two very different sides of the story have been presented: one about the coming of biology, and one about agency and choice. Of course, in historical scholarship, these two perspectives are not normally associated. The indelible legacy of Michel Foucault has ensured that stories about the celebration of agency do not go hand in hand with stories about the coming of biology. Indeed, the new body models developed in the eighteenth century have traditionally been interpreted by historians as a means of enforcing biologically determined subject positions. G. J. Barker-Benfield's is the most extensive of several studies that emphasize the potential inherent within new paradigms to create 'a gendered view of the nerves'.[63] With a similarly Foucauldian hue, Daniel Schafer has identified the advent of the mechanistic paradigm with the medicalization and pathologization of old age. Traditionally then, the body models of Boerhaave and Haller have been interpreted as having the potential to restrict rather than empower. It is second nature now for historians to see biology and agency as forces diametrically opposed, but this opposition does not appear entirely appropriate for a history of the eighteenth-century aging body.

Of course much can be accounted for by differences between theory and practice. In purely theoretical and philosophical terms, the advent of the mechanistic body as the dominant contemporary paradigm for conceptualizing body function offered a profound reformulation for the concept of aging. Although it is anachronistic to say so, the body models formulated by Boerhaave and Haller provided a 'biological' explanation for physical decline over the life course, for they located a nexus of cause and effect within the body which could account for the manifestations of physical aging. The descriptions provided by Boerhaave and Haller were undeniably more 'scientific', more internally focused, and less overtly dependent on the macrocosm. I have argued that the mechanistic physiologists did in fact conceive of something akin to our modern notions of an aging process, for the aging machine functioned on its own terms, and might be considered a discrete biological entity. Furthermore, both physiologists made explicit recognition of the fact that aging was a lifelong process, definitive of human experience, and intrinsic to the very make up of the corporeal frame. The advent of the mechanistic paradigm did present a step towards the theoretical biologization of aging – but only in theory.

This paradigm shift looks very different when surveyed in practical terms. The greatest legacy of the new paradigm to eighteenth-century English culture was the legitimation of agency and self-control. Mechanism provided a new, scientific, secular rationale for endorsing the power of the individual agent over the body and its operations. It provided rules through which the body could be known and controlled; for in mechanistic idiom, even emotional experience could be reduced to mechanical cause and effect. Mechanism was to shine a spotlight on the apparent malleability of the length and pace of life, and the subjectivity of physical aging.

In Chapter 2, I argued that aging, in the eighteenth century, was still considered to happen from the outside in. In reality, neither the mechanistic body nor the sensible body offered any great challenge to this interpretation. Even in the works of Boerhaave and Haller, aging was still considered a largely external phenomenon. They may have provided more scientific descriptions for what went on beneath the skin of the aging machine, but this did not stop them from looking outwards, or appreciating that aging was largely a matter of contingency and choice. New machines ran on the old combination of Non-naturals. In fact, if anything, these new paradigms only enforced the importance of contingency and the outside world. Machines wore out depending on how they were used, what they consumed, how they thought, where they lived. Sensibility was essentially a doctrine based on the acute sensitivity of the sensory system to emotional stimuli in the outside world. Although it might be rationalized rather differently, the aging machine was just as porous as the old humoral body. When it came to the content of advice about the aging body therefore, there is little difference between the advice offered by Floyer and the advice offered by Buchan.

Indeed, the notion of functional exhaustion – the idea that the body 'wore out' by use – did not have to be conveyed through the mechanical idiom. Floyer's vision of the aging body was as much a product of subjective experience or wear and tear as the aging machine. Underwriting Floyer's teachings was a belief that length of human life was essentially a product of the pace at which it is lived, or used up. In *Medicina Gerocomica,* his advice was all about regulating pace or body time: he explained how the body can be used carefully and slowly; how the very mechanisms which engender the body's decay can be slowed down, and how aging may be retarded and longevity achieved. Floyer's core mantra was the need to keep the pulse within compass, particularly to avoid any 'increase' in frequency, as a hasty pulse bespoke a hasty circulation: indicating that the body was being used too fast and hastening the individual towards death.[64] For Floyer, the pulse acted as a life speedometer. He even had a specific 'pulse watch' – a bespoke timepiece – made in order that he could measure it with the utmost accuracy.[65] So although Floyer preferred not to describe the body in the current ideology of the machine, he advocated managing it by using one. What separates writers in terms of their idiom and approach is overshadowed by common recognition that bodies wear out at the rate at which they are used, and this depended a great deal on personal choice. Agency was the common feature of writing about the aging body in eighteenth-century England, whether it was understood as an aging machine, a passionate expressive object, or lamp of life.

4 SOCIETY AND SOCIABILITY: CHEERFULNESS

Introduction

The previous chapter identified the aging body as a particular site for self-control. Thanks to contemporary understandings of body function, it was possible to imagine an aging body extraordinarily pliant to the will. Furthermore, the new body languages of mechanism and (particularly) sensibility emphasized the importance of mental activity and sensory stimulation in bodily management. Emotional experience, medical writers cautioned, could be especially abrasive for the aging body, particularly for those of delicate nerves. This chapter examines the psychosomatic aspect of body management in more detail. It describes how, via a rhetoric of cheerfulness, sociable interaction and positive thinking were championed as the potential solutions for physical aging.

Here the aging body is not just considered as a flesh and blood problem to be solved, but as a site for self-fashioning, and a place for creating modes of socially acceptable behaviour and practice. The social dimension of corporeality has been a fertile area for historical research, and an established literature has done much to connect ideas in medical and philosophical literature to those about conduct, deportment and sociability. Historians have recognized how paradigmatic shifts in philosophy and medicine informed socially acceptable behaviour and practice, and have emphasized the importance of medical texts in mediating notions of bodily expression and societal interaction.[1] Thanks to the endeavours of historians of both eighteenth-century medicine and eighteenth-century culture, we now have a considerable grasp of the social and even political value of body language and self-control in Enlightenment society. The material body, particularly the 'passionate emotional language of the body' in such enterprises was absolutely central.[2] Passion, body language, sentiment and self-control were all means of self definition in eighteenth-century England; and each had their own language or 'visual code', to use the words of Alan McKenzie.[3] As Renate Brosch explains, 'the body language of words, tones, accents and gestures' in eighteenth-century England 'was understood to be a medium by which civility was demonstrated, and also the means by which the several strata of society were to be differentiated'.[4]

Perhaps no aspect of differentiation has received more attention than the culture or 'cult' of sensibility. From the beginning of the eighteenth century, the term 'sensibility' came to be imbued with considerable cultural significance, taking on associations beyond its literal denotation of nervous response. In the words of Joseph Roach, 'sensibility' came to suggest

> a capacity or inherent disposition: the readiness to respond to stimuli, the capacity for emotion as distinct from cognition or will, sensitivity to the pathetic in art or literature or to the feelings of others. [5]

John Mullan's *Sentiment and Sociability: The Language of Feeling in the Eighteenth Century*, has demonstrated how medical writings concerned with nervous disorders – produced in a steady flow between about 1720 and 1770 – shared with novels and philosophical works a 'language of feeling' based on the psycho-perceptual schemes formulated by Newton and Locke. As Mullan explains, eighteenth-century writers 'discover in their writings a sociability which is dependant on the communication of passions and sentiments'.[6] Similarly, Robert Markley has written of 'a form of moral self-promotion' that manifested itself in a variety of genres: the novel, moral conduct books, philosophical discourse and medical literature.[7] 'What unites these disparate forms', Markley writes, 'is their authors' ideological preoccupation with emerging middle-class virtues of sensitivity, generosity, natural sympathy, health, and physical beauty.'[8] In short, the ability to comprehend the body as a sensitive, reactive mechanism was at the source of dominant cultural theories of society: a 'peculiar intensity of emotional expression' that William Reddy has denominated nothing less than a unique historical 'regime'.[9]

As yet the specific contribution of the aging body to this regime of expressiveness remains unexplored. Throughout this chapter I attempt to fill that gap, and to demonstrate the singular significance of the aging body in informing contemporary notions of sociability and the forces of Enlightenment society. Above all, I wish to draw attention to the previously unacknowledged role of 'cheerfulness' in the Enlightenment regime. In eighteenth-century England, cheerfulness was a means of managing the aging body. It was a way of exercising agency over the aging process via the mind and via society. Although being cheerful in old age had been considered appropriate since Aristotle, the meaning and value of cheerfulness took on a new significance in the medico-commercial culture under examination here. Cheerfulness was also an important part of Enlightenment culture and sociability in its own right. It had its own ideology and its own rhetoric, through which managing the aging body could be discussed as an endeavour with sociable, social and even political ends.

This chapter begins by introducing the concept of cheerfulness in an eight-eenth-century context, looking at both its etymology and a number of essays, tracts and literary pieces that address its meaning and power. It then looks at how cheerfulness was said to 'work' in medical advice. The final section of the chapter presents some observations about the value of cheerfulness as a force within society, positioning the idea in the context of contemporary theories of 'sympathy' and emotional communication.

Cheerfulness

To eighteenth-century readers, cheerfulness was a concept that was rich, ready and significant. Rather like that key eighteenth-century term, 'politeness', 'cheerfulness' had distinct social and moral values that have been washed out of our understanding of the word today. Cheerfulness could convey notions of psychosomatic calmness, freedom from passionate turmoil, closeness to God, humanistic appreciation, civic virtue, sociability and self-control. And, on top of these associations, it had a definite physical – even medical – value. Cheerfulness had a direct power over the body and a specific value for health, almost as if it could be imagined as a material essence. It was in this sense in particular that it had real power over physical aging. In order to get a sense of its unique semantic potential, it is necessary to look at the both the etymology of cheerfulness and some of its uses in various eighteenth-century contexts – examples from diction-aries, essays, tracts, literary pieces and advertisements – that give a sense of its resonance in the eighteenth-century imagination.

Nowadays, cheerfulness – defined by the *Oxford English Dictionary* as 'noticeably happy and optimistic' – seems a rather insipid and vacuous word and unsurprisingly its use is not favoured. Today it conveys a state of mind, an out-look; a mental property; a characteristic way of engaging with the world. Yet our eighteenth-century forebears would be more attuned to some of its now for-gotten *physical* meanings. The word is descended from the Old French 'chiere', meaning 'face', and the Latin 'cara', or Greek 'kara', both of which mean 'head'. In its original sense, then, cheerfulness referred directly to the face itself and only by extension to that face's expression or mood. Later it took on the specific meaning of a positive mood.

By the mid eighteenth-century, when Johnson came to compile his *Diction-ary*, cheerfulness was still definable in these distinctly physical, tangible ways. Johnson opened his definition by explaining that the word was to be understood as combining the French meaning of the physical face, or as he put it, 'air of the countenance', and the Spanish concept of cheer as entertainment and nourish-ment: the food and fun that we occasionally refer to antiquatedly as 'good cheer'. As Johnson noted, the idea of 'cheerfulness' was replete with both associations.

'It seems to have, in English, some relation to both these senses', he wrote. The physical and remedial qualities of cheer and cheerfulness were further endorsed by Johnson's next reference, which was to physic. Under his definition of a 'cheerer', Johnson quoted a maxim from Queen Anne's physician, Sir William Temple: 'Saffron is the fastest and most simple cordial, the greatest reviver of the heart, and cheerer of the spirits.'[10] Cheering was a physical act which could be carried out on the body, and which could affect subcutaneous body mechanisms (it was possible to make reference to a 'cheerful' circulation).[11] Hence eighteenth-century cheerfulness was something more somatic and physical than we might gather from our concept today.

Cheerfulness had a distinct social value and currency in eighteenth-century England. Essayists and correspondents saw cheerfulness as a topic of worthy consideration. Maxims, essays, conduct books and writings on the passions identified cheerfulness as beneficial not only at the personal but also the social level. To the individual body and mind it brought an unflappable calmness and ease, but it also brought sociability and improved social interaction. In some contexts it could even represent Christian, civic or moral virtue. Perhaps the most often quoted and plagiarized eighteenth-century essay on cheerfulness was by Joseph Addison.[12] In his *Spectator* piece 'On Cheerfulness', Addison sought to consider cheerfulness in three contexts: 'with Regard to ourselves, to those we converse with, and to the great Author of our Being'.[13] The significance of cheerfulness was not, in short, confined to the unit of the individual. Its values were socially improving and spiritually and morally defensible.

Cheerfulness represented an ideal stasis; it signified a body and mind uninterrupted by human folly and the emotional demands of everyday life. In the classical framework for comprehending health, the passions were considered invested with a power to discompose and deviate body and mind from their natural, stable course. Passionate upheaval was unhealthy, and ideally one should strive for calmness in order to preserve health. As one author of an early-century work entitled *A Natural History of the Passions* (1701), narrated,

> every man living find[s] his spirit sometimes calm and serene, sometimes agitated and ruffled more or less by the winds and tempests of passions raised within him.[14]

Cheerfulness represented the former predicament, what the author called a 'halcyon state' of body and mind: natural, ideal poise. Cheerfulness was like a protective layer: it removed proneness and lessened irritability. As Godwin explained at the end of the century, 'even bodily pain loses much of its sting when it is encountered by a cheerful, a composed, and a determined spirit'.[15] Cheerfulness promoted health because the body was more tranquil, more guarded against attacks, and therefore more able to carry on steady function which led to health, prevented disease and aided long life. Like any classically educated gentleman, Addison knew that in Aristotelian–Galenic philosophy, states of mind had tangible, quantifiable influences beneath the skin, and he was keen to state that the most visible value of cheerfulness was its physical effect on the body. 'In the first Place', he revealed, cheerfulness was 'the best Promoter of Health'.[16] 'CHEARFULNESS' wrote Addison,

> bears the same friendly Regard to the Mind as to the Body; it banishes all anxious Care and Discontent, sooths and composes the Passions, and keeps the Soul in a perpetual Calm.[17]

Whether it was mental, somatic or divine, this 'perfect Calm' had a real power to preserve health and prolong life; cheerfulness begat longevity.

This specific, tangible power of cheerfulness was highlighted in devotional works. Richard Steele's *Discourse on Old Age* argued that 'a cheerful Heart, a sober Diet, and moderate Exercise, may defer old Age for a Time'.[18] Steele equated cheerfulness with the temperance, abstention and asceticism characteristic of traditional regimen, and suggested that cheerfulness had temperate, sobering effects upon the body. Noticeably, Steele located its presence in the heart rather than the head, a further reminder that cheerfulness was not, in the eighteenth-century imagination, necessarily a mental quality. In a section of his *Enquiry After Happiness* (1734), devoted specifically to 'The Ways of Prolonging Life', the minister Richard Lucas determined to demonstrate exactly why 'the chearfulness of the mind has a very propitious ... influence upon the life of man'.[19] Venturing in to physiological terminology, he explained that,

> the contentment of the mind preserves the balsam of the blood, and the pleasure of it enlarges the heart, raises the spirits, actuates and invigorates all our powers; so that when the mind shines serene and bright, it seems to impart a new warmth and new life to the body, a new spring and new verdure to this earth. On the contrary, a diseas'd mind does, as it were, scatter its contagion through the body; discontent and melancholy, sour the blood and clog the spirits; envy pines away, and passion frets and wears out our strength and life. **In few words, the intimate conjunction** between the mind and body; and so close is the dependence of the latter upon the former, that the face of interiour nature does evidently vary, wither or flourish, according to that variety of weather it makes in the sky above it, as the mind smiles or lowers upon it.[20]

Summarizing his philosophy, Lucas had opened the *Enquiry* professing that it was 'obvious and manifest to every one' that 'life' depended upon 'three things: the chearfulness of the mind, the health of the body, and a favourable providence of God'.[21] Here, cheerfulness forms part of the tripartite recipe for 'life' itself: it is a very principle of vitality and longevity.

The therapeutic and physical value of cheerfulness in the popular imagination is suggested by the frequency of its inclusion in titles, headings and advertisements in printed material on health and longevity. 'Cheerfulness' is frequently to be found married to concepts of 'health' in these contexts, suggesting that the word was something of a slogan for physical soundness and holistic well-being. The sub-title to John Hill's *Virtues of Sage, in Lengthening Human Life*, was *Rules to Attain Old Age in Health and Cheerfulness*. Late-century newspapers confirm this habitual coupling; a number of advertisements for tinctures and medicines entwined concepts of cheerfulness and health, or simply included 'cheerfulness' in their text. The 'Genuine TINCTURE of HEALTH VALERIAN' for 'Nervous Disorders, and Hysteric Complaints' (a potion 'faithfully prepared' according to the manuscript recipe of the prolific Dr Hill) promised that the first symptoms of recovery would be 'serenity and cheerfulness'.[22] Another proffered remedy for 'nervous disorders of every kind', the 'Samaritan Restorative', claimed to furnish its consumers with 'cheerfulness, and every presage of lasting Health'.[23] The 'celebrated cordial balm of Gilead' offered the exact same combination.[24] In these advertisements, cheerfulness appears to signify the quiet mind that proceeded from, accompanied or begot a body in good working order. As is perhaps suggested by the specific connection with nervous disorders, cheerfulness appears to be a term of especial significance within the language and culture of sensibility. Other products aimed in particular at improving the circulation offered 'cheerfulness of mind', and the advertisement for 'Aromatic Lozenges of Steel' associated cheerfulness with a more robust, active notion of physical function, offering 'health and vigour to the debilitated frame', and 'cheerfulness and animation in the mind'.[25]

Whereas it may seem intuitive to think that a sound body is accompanied by a sense of pleasant mental ease, the use of 'cheerfulness' in such contexts represents more than a trite or empty turn of phrase about psychosomatic well-being. Although it may have figured within contemporary parlance as a little-considered cliché, or in contemporary advertising as a well-worn commercial catchphrase, its associations with health were more serious, somatic and integral. In his *Old Man's Guide*, Hill defined cheerfulness as 'the natural offspring of health'.[26] Cheyne reckoned that the '*Wisdom, the Art, and Perfection of Physic*', was 'to make a Man live cheerful and easy, without Pain or Disease'.[27] The particular frequency of its use suggests that to the writers and readers of eighteenth-century medical literature it had a special signifying power: the ability to conjure images of physical soundness. As such it may be seen as quasi-official medical terminology.

Like politeness, the term 'cheerfulness' could represent an entire behavioural code, the benefits of which were to be reaped at a societal level. Cheerfulness and politeness had much in common. Cheerfulness certainly involved 'pleasing in company', for the particular calmness it engendered could be considered especially appropriate for polite, sociable interaction. 'When joy is settled into a habit, or flows from a placid temper of mind, *formed to please, and be pleased*, it is called Gaiety, Good Humour, or Chearfulness', explained John Bethum in his discourse on the passions.[28] As the arbiter of taste and champion of middle-class ethics of restraint, it was this socializing, civilizing element of cheerfulness that Addison was particularly keen to endorse. Dovetailing nicely with his philosophy was the educative and improving potential inherent in cheerfulness. For Addison, cheerfulness was a force that might be harnessed for the benefit of society. Outwardly it signalled composure and was antithetical to unchecked enthusiastic or emotional display. He had, he insisted, 'always preferred cheerfulness to mirth'.[29] Cheerfulness appeared to Addison to be a quality especially fitting for polite civility; it was, he wrote, a state of mind emphatically fitting for the polite citizen in 'the present State of Humanity'.[30] The cultivation of cheerfulness definitely fell within the remit of those aspiring to socially acceptable 'polite' behaviour.

It was impossible to consider the physical benefits of cheerfulness without conceding that this perfect serenity was the product and proof of a soul close to God. Cheerfulness had a spiritual dimension. Searching for titles including the word 'cheerfulness' in the British Library catalogue brings up scores of works connected to contented piety and devotion. Yet cheerfulness had a particular, eighteenth-century resonance that conveyed far more than religious observance. Cheerfulness represented a *socially turned* breed of piety; one characterized not by sombre devotion but by healthy, hygienic, social interaction and pleasing levity. It was the kind of Christian virtue that had an implicit social value, as Laurence Sterne was keen to illustrate. Berating too grave a sense of religion, in his own essay 'On Chearfulness', Sterne reminded his readers that 'Plato and Seneca ... thought that a sense of chearfulness and joy should ever be encouraged in children, from their infancy'.[31] This was not 'only on account of their healths, but as productive of true virtue', he explained, for 'Chearfulness, even to gaiety, is consonant with every species of virtue, and practice of religion'.[32] Cheerfulness could be an outward signifier of moral integrity, a habit that was itself productive of virtue and devotion.

For some writers, there was something deeply natural and genuinely human about being in a state of cheerfulness. Writers often gave the sense that it accompanied purity, spiritual, moral, somatic and moral. For Addison, cheerfulness represented an idyllic and benign human state. It suggested a contented awareness and acquiescence within the divine scheme of things, the beauty of which might be experienced 'inwardly' by the cheerful individual. As Addison saw it,

> an inward Chearfulness is an implicit Praise and Thanksgiving to Providence under all its Dispensations: It is a Kind of Acquiescence in the State wherein we are placed, and a secret Approbation of the Divine Will in his Conduct towards Man.[33]

Rationality could also be reflected and begotten by cheerfulness. In this sense, cheerfulness represented an ability to master oneself, and apex of disciplined self-control. This was a key part of Addison's formulation:

> The Man who is possessed of this excellent Frame of Mind, is not only easy in his
> Thoughts, but perfect Master of all the Powers and Faculties of his Soul; his Imagi-
> nation is always clear, and his Judgement undisturbed; his Temper is even and
> unruffled, whether in Action or in Solitude; he comes with a Relish to all those
> Goods which Nature has provided for him, tastes all the Pleasures of the Creation
> which are poured about him, and does not feel the full Weight of those accidental
> Evils which may befall him.[34]

Embodying explicit connections between spirituality, morality and health, cheerfulness serves to remind us of the multi-dimensionality of well-being in eighteenth-century England. In the words of Philip Rieder, 'health' was 'not just a question concerning the body, or at least not the body as we know it today'.[35] Cheerfulness might have manifested itself on the body in certain specific and beneficial ways, but at root it was a higher presence that could account for these manifestations. In this sense, cheerfulness served to represent the inherent spiritual, Christian dimension of bodily management. Of course, the overweening presence of the body spiritual continued to pervade the most authoritative and the most popular writings on the aging body, most obviously those of Cheyne and Wesley. As the devout doctor was careful to keep reminding his readers, the physical benefits of devotion were enormous. 'The *Love of God*', he wrote, which 'by the unspeakable Joy, and perfect Calm, Serenity and Tranquility it gives the Mind, becomes the most *powerful* of all the *Means* of *Health* and *Long Life*.'[36] Cheerfulness might be described as oneness with God; a cheerful body was one that reflected and acquiesced in His omnipotence and benevolence. Ideas about the real power of cheerfulness over flesh and blood embody very traditional anxieties about spiritual probity reflected in the physical body. However, the power of cheerfulness did not only depend on traditional anxieties or the old ways of thinking. As will be discussed in the following section, although cheerfulness had played a role within medical thought since the ancients, its power and unique contemporary significance was even more resonant when expressed through the new body languages of mechanism and sensibility.

Medical Advice

In the medical writings of eighteenth-century England, cheerfulness was considered a specific, signifying concept with its own physical manifestations. It was described as a particular psychosomatic state that provided an antidote to the aging body, a means of self-preservation against physical decline. In the eyes of eighteenth-century doctors, cheerfulness was conceived to have direct, quantifiable and categorical relationships with the very vital functions that regulated life and decay – in particular the pace of the circulation. When Buchan wrote that, 'whoever would live to a good old age, must be good humoured and cheerful', it was because, as he went on to explain, 'cheerfulness and mirth quicken the circulation, and promote all the secretions, whereas sadness and profound thought never fail to retard them.'[37] Cheerfulness carried an intrinsic somatic value, and in medical advice the very mention of cheerfulness brought visions of a beneficial bodily function. The medical and social reformer, Dr Thomas Beddoes, writing his *Lecture Introductory to a Course of Popular Instruction of the Constitution and Management of the Human Body*, in 1797, was able to assume that cheerfulness *was* entirely synonymous with bodily healthiness. 'Some observer of mankind has remarked that it is better to be born to a cheerful temper than to ten thousand a year', he wrote, progressing immediately to explain his meaning thus:

> I can conceive that organs, pleasantly performing their functions through most of the seven stages of life, are of as much value to the possessor, as accomplishments capable, for some few fleeting moments, of enrapturing ten thousand beaux. [38]

'A cheerful temper' was tantamount to a body destined for longevity. The connection was implicit: 'cheerfulness' just meant health and long life. In the medical imagination, cheerfulness was almost terminology; a synonym for health and the psychosomatic prescription for longevity. New body models and psycho-perceptual schemes could now contribute to and legitimize the endorsement of a mind-over-matter approach to the management of aging, and explain how – physically, subcutaneously – the right sorts of thinking, and the right sort of mental stimulation, had tangible, quantifiable effects on vital processes which brought about decline. Cheerfulness represented the specific psychosomatic recipe that would, in the eyes of eighteenth-century physicians, slow down the pace of bodily decay. In terms of the aging body, therefore, cheerfulness was *the* aspirational quality *par excellence*, and was championed as a significant achievement of mind over matter.

By extolling the health benefits of cheerfulness for the aging body, writers of medical advice were drawing upon a long established medical tradition that acknowledged the power of passionate experience to affect the body. The mental-corporeal continuum envisaged by Galenic physiology had ensured that the 'passions' had always played a central role in accounting for physical decline within the medical tradition. Of course, the 'passions' were one of the six tabulated 'Non-naturals' along with air, food, sleep, exercise and evacuations: these were the forces of nature that needed to be mediated for a long and healthy life. In the Galenic idiom, mental activity blended seamlessly with physical experience to produce identical results. Emotions, therefore, worked in the same way as more tangible 'cures' for the body, and passions could be equated with other Non-naturals as a result of their common effects on the body. As Floyer had taken for granted in his *Medicina Gerocomica*, 'cold Air, cold Baths, cold Diet ... cold Cloaths, cold Beds', might have exactly the same result as the 'cooling

Passions of Fear and Sadness'.[39] Specific emotional experiences had always been thought to hasten or deter the onset of old age, and this Floyer rehearsed for his readers. 'Immoderate Cares and Passions, especially Sorrow, hasten old Age', he explained.[40] 'Envy, Ambition, Covetousness, Anger, do decay the Body; but Hope, Love, Joy, are Prolongers of our Lives by their Influence on the Humours.'[41]

Despite the waning of the Galenic scheme, the passions continued as staple fare in medical advice, and could now be said to work via the new models of body function. Passions were just as central for the mechanistic body as they were for the humoral body, and even more so for those who championed sensibility. Within the new schemes, established associations remained. It was the same passions of joy, love and hope that were generally thought beneficial for aging bodies, and the same broadly negative ones that were described to have detrimental effects. Within the established configuration, cheerfulness was not often singled out as a recognizable, independent 'passion', but was often equated with the more oft quoted 'joy', and sometimes it was contrasted with 'mirth'. Traditionally, 'joy' was considered a beneficial corporeal fillip that roused the physical motions. At the end of the seventeenth century, Descartes translated these same effects into mechanical idiom. In the ninety-ninth article of his *Passions de l'Ame*, he qualified the effects of joy thus:

> In Joy, that the pulse is even and quicker than ordinary, but not so strong, nor so great as in Love, and that a man feels a pleasant heat, which is not onely in the breast, but spreads it self over all the exteriour parts of the body, with the blood, which is seen to flow abundantly thither: and the mean while he sometimes loses his appetite, because the digestion is lesse than usuall.[42]

As the physical effects of cheerfulness were comparable to those of joy, it was seen to have a particularly beneficial effect in rousing and stimulating the body and revitalizing its functions. As the anonymous author of one mid-century text, *The Best and Easiest Method of Preserving Uninterrupted Health to Extreme Old Age* (1748), explained,

> joy and Chearfulness promote Perspiration, by exciting the Motion of our Fluids; they give a free Admission to our Spirits, and enervate the whole System of the Fibres; they thin the Juices, and cause all our Secretions which depend upon a regular Circulation of the Blood to be justly perform'd.[43]

Although joy and cheerfulness were often discussed together, cheerfulness had a certain qualification that made it particularly suitable for the aging body. Unlike joy, cheerfulness was never vehement or harmful; it was always benign, whereas excessive joy might bubble over uncontrollably. An over-enthusiastic expression of joy had its own term: 'mirth'. Mirth, although acceptable and indeed appropriate in youth, might be too strong and harmful for weaker or aged constitutions.

As John Hill explained in his *Old Man's Guide,* it was 'ease', 'calmness', 'temperance' and 'cheerfulness' that were the appropriate qualities to characterize 'the advanced period considered here':[44]

> Joy is, in a violent degree, as hurtful as the other passions: it hurries the circulation vehemently, and irregularly; it exhausts the spirits; and has occasioned sudden death. It is a violence of youth; it belongs to that period of life; that can bear it; and to that let us leave it. Let the old man be as the Quakers in this point; always cheerful but never merry.[45]

The particular qualification that made cheerfulness especially suitable for the aging body was also that which made it ideal for polite sociability. As Addison had emphasized in the *Spectator,* a sedate, steady cheerfulness was infinitely preferable to effusive displays of mirth. Cheerfulness was impossible to experience in excess; it was characterized by moderation. During the eighteenth century – a period characterized by its own emphasis on doctrines of politeness and refinement – the endorsement of cheerfulness was to become particularly opportune. Advice about managing the aging body blended with more general endorsements of the qualities suitable for polite behaviour. By extension, management of the aging body became a visible means of exhibiting behaviours that conformed to hegemonic behavioural codes of politeness and restraint. At this particular historical moment, management of the aging body and polite sociability shared a rhetoric of cheerfulness. These two enterprises could unite to a common, improving purpose, underlining the value of aging body management to a progressive and polite Enlightenment society.

The connection between ease and longevity was deeply entrenched, perhaps intuitive. However, envisaging the body as a machine allowed the positive effects of cheerfulness to become more quantifiable and real.[46] Cheerfulness was called upon with repeated frequency in the language of the new physiological paradigms. Indeed, it was remarkably well suited to it. The aging machine could now be said to benefit from cheerfulness because of its quantifiable effect on the pace and regulation of vital functions. Cheerfulness prevented the body from wearing out. A volatile, passion-wrought mind was as detrimental to the body as any kind of physical exertion, and certainly prohibitive of longevity. As Addison explained in his defence of cheerfulness as a 'Promoter of Health', passionate yearnings might not be so visible as physical stress, but they were all the more dangerous for their being imperceptible:

> Repinings and secret Murmurings of the Heart give imperceptible Strokes to those delicate Fibres of which the vital Parts are composed, and wear out the Machine insensibly.[47]

In mechanistic ideology, a person likely to achieve longevity was known by a body and mind untroubled by too much motion, or use. As characterized by Boerhaave, longevity could be achieved by slowness and calmness of function. The somatic signifiers of longevity were,

> a slow, large, full easy, even Respiration ... a slow, large, full, equal, strong, constant or steady Pulse of the Arteries ... a slow Provocation to Stool ... moderate Labour, a dull Genius and not too violent Motion of the Mind or Body.[48]

In mechanical and somatic terms, cheerfulness was synonymous with slowness. It promoted longevity because it made the aging machine function move slowly and carefully. Haller identified cheerfulness as a specific indicator of the moderation and mildness that characterized optimal function and which would augur longevity:

> Some prerogatives of long life seem to be sobriety, at least a moderate and not very rich diet; a mild behaviour; a mind not endowed with very great vivacity, but cheerful, and little subject to care.[49]

It was not only bodily tardiness that was desirable for longevity, but also mental slowness – even to the extent of dimness. Despite all its connections with piety and virtue, cheerfulness could also represent intellectual slowness – a kind of blissful ignorance. In medical advice, 'cheerfulness' is often defined as the antithesis to intense thought and introversion, and the readiness with which cheerfulness is set up as a contrast to self-indulgent introverted intellectual activity is striking. Sometimes, cheerfulness acts a happy check on an otherwise dangerously errant mind. At others, cheerfulness is contrasted to intellectual activity *tout court*, to the point even where ignorance is esteemed valuable.

Buchan was certainly sceptical about a group of people he referred to as 'the Studious'. In a scathing sweep he pronounced them universally unfit for longevity. 'Intense thought is so destructive to health', Buchan wrote,

> that few instances can be produced of studious persons who live to an extreme old age ... Man is evidently not formed for continual thought more than for perpetual action, and would be as soon worn out by the one as by the other.[50]

In order to confirm this sentiment, Buchan called upon 'Chearfulness' and its subcutaneous effects, juxtaposing it not only against 'sadness', but also against 'profound thought', and recommending therefore 'a degree of thoughtlessness' as 'necessary' for health and longevity.[51] Cheerfulness or 'cheerful company' was often presented as the antidote to the kind of mental habits or intellectual exertion that was physically abrasive. For those who were in danger of wearing themselves out through intellectual exertion, cheerfulness offered a therapeutic refuge, as Buchan explained:

Perpetual thinkers, as they are called, seldom think to much purpose. Such people, in a course of years, generally become quite stupid, and exhibit a melancholy proof how readily the greatest blessings may be abused. Thought, like all other things, when carried to extreme, becomes a vice. Hence nothing can afford a greater proof of wisdom than for a man frequently and seasonably to unbend his mind. This may always be done by cheerful company, active diversions, music, or the like.[52]

As he demonstrated in his *Enquiry after Happiness* (1734), Richard Lucas thought it was common knowledge that cheerfulness led to longevity:

I believe, we may safely pronounce, that generally, such live longest, who either think very little, or whose thoughts are always calm and cheerful; such who are stupid, and have no passions; or are wise and good, and have none but such as are regular and delightful.[53]

Correlations between cheerfulness, longevity, slowness and dull-wittedness pervade medical advice. Intellectual activity is treated with a certain disdain, for cheerfulness seems incompatible with cerebral and academic pursuits. 'In order to acquire and maintain a green old Age', wrote the German doctor Johann Friedrich Cohausen in his *Hermippus Redivivus: or, The Sage's Triumph over Old Age and the Grave*, of 1743, 'there is nothing so requisite as Chearfulness of Mind, which can never be secured, if we meditate much on abstruse subjects.'[54] In a Boswellian anecdote, we encounter the implied assumption that cheerfulness was opposite to intense philosophical meditation. Boswell described how Dr Johnson had run into an old friend from his university days, a man by the name of Mr Edwards. After some conversation, Edwards duly remarked on Johnson's renowned genius, contrasting it to his own proclivities:

You are a philosopher, Dr. Johnson. I have tried too in my time to be a philosopher; but, I don't know how, cheerfulness was always breaking in.[55]

The sentiment behind such an expression may strike the modern reader as somewhat glib, perhaps even disrespectful – at face value Edwards seems to be implying that Johnson is a moody, introverted scholar. However, it must be supposed that when uttered it was intended to convey a more definite contrast, a difference perhaps resulting from varying degrees of nervous pliability.

The juxtaposition between cheerfulness and abstruse meditation was a device loaded with potential for discussing aging and the sensible body, both in medical advice itself and in the wider discussion of this 'cult'. According to the philosophy of nervous sensibility, an individual's intellectual capacity was considered dependent on the structure of their nerves. In Cheyne's *English Malady* (1733), a work devoted to nervous disorders, he had divided humankind into three classes on the basis of the speed, agility and depth of their perceptions. 'The common Division of Mankind into *Quick Thinkers*, *Slow Thinkers*, and *No*

Thinkers', he wrote, 'is not without Foundation in Nature and true Philosophy.'[56] Quick thinkers were likely to be persons of agile imaginations, easily moved, sensitive and – importantly in this context – somewhat prone to introspection. Such persons were not likely to achieve longevity, as their errant minds could wear out the body. Part of Cheyne's remit in advising such persons – among which he counted himself – involved providing useful directions for taming an errant mind. Cheerfulness featured heavily in his advice:

> It seems to me absolutely impossible, without such a Help to keep the Mind easy, and prevent its wearing out the Body, as the Sword does the Scarbbard; it is no matter what it is, provided it be but a *Hobby-Horse* and an Amusement, and stop the Current of reflexion and intense Thinking which Persons of weak Nerves are aptest to run into … And therefore ingenious Flattering, easy and agreeable Amusements, and Intervals of No-thinking and *Swiss-Meditation*, (as it is maliciously called) is as necessary for such, as Sleep to the Weary, or Meat to the Hungry, else the Spring will break, and the Sword wear out the Scabbard. *Study* of difficult and intricate Matters will infallibly do Hurt. *Reading* must be light, entertaining, and diverting, as well as Food.[57]

Within this idiom, cheerfulness came to represent a means of overcoming the limitations of a delicate physiology; a state that offered respite from an overly sensitive, artistic temperament. The self-confessed 'Man of Feeling', Samuel Johnson, defined 'cheerfulness' in his *Dictionary* with all these attendant associations. Cheerfulness for Johnson was the opposite of the blues; it was 'freedom from gloominess' or 'freedom from dejection'. It was through 'cheerfulness', he suggested, that men of his persuasion might find 'respite' from their psychological and intellectual tendencies.

It was this particular nuance that the doctor and poet Mark Akenside acclaimed in his poem, the 'Hymn to Cheerfulness' (1788). Akenside's knowledge of nervous aetiology equipped him rather well for handling the subject. He had taken medical degrees from the universities of Edinburgh and Leiden, and on his return to England occupied a succession of important medical posts, including principal physician at St Thomas's Hospital, assistant physician at the school of Christ's Hospital, and physician-in-ordinary to Queen Charlotte. Yet as well as being a successful physician and medical writer, Akenside was (in the opinion of Samuel Johnson) a poet of considerable ability. His first major work, *The Pleasures of Imagination*, a philosophical poem in which he popularized Addison's ideas from the *Spectator*, appeared in 1744, and went through three further authorized editions before the end of the year.[58] In another of Akenside's literary publications – one which similarly combined the influence of his medically-informed imagination with aesthetic subjects – Akenside wrote of the particular value of cheerfulness. *Odes on Several Subjects*, of 1754, a collection of ten lyrics, contained the aforementioned *Hymn*.[59]

Referencing the language of delicate nerves and emotional strain, Akenside described a picture of the vulnerability of the acutely sensible body, and its dangerous propensity to be moved by storms both meteorological and emotional. The *Hymn* began with an image of a dark, oppressive evening that 'Tear[s] the frail texture of my veins' and 'renew[s] mind's oppressive gloom'.[60] Faced with such a prospect, he implores the reader, rhetorically,

> is there in nature no kind power
> To sooth affliction's lonely hour?
> To blunt the edge of dire disease,
> And teach these wintry shades to please?[61]

In such a situation, Akenside imagines that the antidote to such gloominess and dejection is cheerfulness. In an attempt to 'brighten the dejected scene', he summons an anthropomorphized figure of 'Cheerfulness':

> Come, Cheerfulness, triumphant fair,
> Shine through the hovering cloud of care
> O sweet of language, mild of mien,
> O virtue's friend and pleasure's queen
> Asswage the flames that burn my breast
> Compose my jarring thoughts to rest,
> And while thy gracious gifts I feel,
> My song shall all thy praise reveal.[62]

Demonstrating the ability of cheerfulness to calm the heat of passionate experience, and restore a more mild, composed outlook, Akenside recognizes both the medico-therapeutic value of cheerfulness, and its more aesthetic, social and spiritual resonance. Indeed, the imagined Goddess of 'Cheerfulness', Akenside explains, is the result of a union between male 'Health' and female 'Love'.[63] In Akenside's imagination, cheerfulness is a politeness beneath the skin, the psychosomatic state that enables an outward composure, a pleasing benevolent, virtuous sociability; attuned to pleasures of nature and the imagination. Cheerfulness represents the specific prescription for composure packaged in the idiom of the sensible body. On a more esoteric level, it also establishes the state of 'cheerfulness' as a refuge for persons of weak nerves. Cheerfulness, in this idiom, may be seen as a socially responsible helpline for the artistic temperament: a means of self-mastery.

In the medically inspired writings of eighteenth-century England, then, cheerfulness was a specific, signifying concept with its own physical manifestations. It was described as the particular psychosomatic state that provided an antidote to the aging body, a means of self-preservation against physical decline. Yet this rhetoric of cheerfulness had a far broader significance; self-mastery of the (aging) body achieved through cheerfulness had a definite socio-ethical value. Cheerfulness did not only prevent physical aging, but also produced a body unswayed by passionate experience, socially turned, pious, benevolent, virtuous and carefully policed. It was therefore in tune with the particular, historically specific civic and social values endorsed by dominant contemporary behavioural codes, and it was particularly suited to the new paradigms of bodily function, and the culture of sensibility. As such, cheerfulness had a particular eighteenth-century application, resonance and power. At the end of the century, when the radical philosopher William Godwin came to write his clarion masterwork, it was possible for him to imagine cheerfulness as a specific force of good in society: part of a socio-ethical prescription for improvement and the progress of humankind.

Godwin's controversial *Enquiry Concerning Political Justice* (1793) was a compendious work, best known for its radical philosophy of individualism. Central to this philosophy was Godwin's faith in the progress of the human mind and its omnipotence over matter, and he drew heavily on the nascent 'psychology' of David Hartley to verify his ideas. According to Godwin, it was possible, with the right mental fortitude, to overcome bodily infirmities and disease: 'Indisposition only becomes formidable in proportion as it is seconded by the consent of the mind', 'we are sick and we die, generally speaking, because we consent to suffer these accidents'.[64] With such faith in the 'infinite' qualities of the human mind over flesh, it was perhaps inevitable that Godwin should champion psychosomatic mastery over the aging process. For Godwin, aging was totally a capacity of the self, a matter of choice. People only became old because they changed their thoughts and habits, and it was only as a result of these deliberate changes that the body aged:

> Why is it that a mature man soon loses that elasticity of limb, which characterises the heedless gaiety of youth? Because he desists from youthful habits. He assumes an air of dignity incompatible with the lightness of childish sallies. He is visited and vexed with all the cares that rise out of our mistaken institutions, and his heart is no longer satisfied and gay. Hence his limbs become stiff and unwieldy. This is the forerunner of old age and death.[65]

Godwin's solution was none other than 'chearfulness'. He thought that it might be the means of banishing aging and achieving immortality. It is clear from his descriptions that he assumed cheerfulness to have a physical power over the aging body. Cheerfulness was no mere state of mind; it was a very 'corporeal' issue:

> The first habit favourable to corporeal vigour is chearfulness. Every time that our mind becomes morbid, vacant and melancholy, a certain period is cut off from the length of our lives. Listlessness of thought is the brother of death. But chearfulness gives new life to our frame and circulation to our juices.[66]

Referencing the particular benefit of cheerfulness to the circulation of the blood, Godwin drew upon specific therapeutic ideas outlined in medical literature. He also juxtaposed cheerfulness to morbidity and melancholia (as it often was in the idiom of sensibility). The fact that Godwin was able to draw upon these ideas in 1793 suggests that cheerfulness was established as an accepted trope – and one with especial value for the aging body. It was this semantic richness that Godwin could draw upon to make his eventual, radical claim that cheerfulness might facilitate immortality. He believed he had identified a 'principle of immortality in man' and this 'principle', as he called it, was 'chearfulness, clearness of conception and benevolence'.[67]

Historians have recognized the importance of some of the other concepts that Godwin uses – 'benevolence' and 'sympathy', for example – as key terms in contemporary philosophical enquiry, the intangible 'forces of society' that fascinated eighteenth-century ontologists such as Hume and Smith. What we have not recognized is that when Godwin talked about cultivating 'cheerfulness', he is similarly drawing upon a specific rhetoric which, like sympathy or benevolence, had a very particular contemporary value and relevance. Cheerfulness, in the eighteenth-century imagination, was a concept laden with value, so much so that it could be given a socio-political impulse.

Sociability and the Forces of Society

Cheerfulness and sociability were intrinsically linked. In medical advice, one of the definitive aspects of cheerfulness was that it was something to be sought *in company*. When providing advice about how to alleviate the aging process via cheerfulness, medical writers frequently explained that cheerfulness resulted from pleasant sensory stimulation in pleasing and polite sociable activity. 'Nothing will more effectually contribute towards the Felicity of a *Green Old Age*', Cheyne wrote, 'than innocent and entertaining *Amusements*, engageing and light Studies, and rational *Diversions* in a cheerful and affectionat Society.'[68] Similarly, the anonymous *Eminent Physician* (1729) suggested that 'old People' should 'regale their Minds, by diverting themselves in chearful, pleasant Company'.[69] Within medical advice, the word 'cheerful' functioned as a stamp of approval for habits, pursuits and behaviours characterized by their sociable nature. As Buchan told his readers, 'nothing can afford a greater proof of wisdom for a man frequently and seasonably to unbend his mind ... this may be done by cheerful company, active diversions, music, or the like'.[70] Medical writers were not shy in spelling out what was and what was not cheerful, and often they presented their readers with a simple choice between self-indulgent introversion and sociable interaction. Buchan was emphatic:

> whoever would live to a good old age, must be good humoured and chearful. This indeed
> is not altogether in our own power; yet our temper of mind, as well as actions, depends
> greatly upon ourselves. We can either think of agreeable or disagreeable objects, as we
> chuse; we can go into chearful or melancholy company; we can mingle in the amuse-
> ments and offices of life, or sit still and brood over our calamities. These, and many such
> things, are certainly in our power, and from these the mind generally takes its cast.[71]

Cheerfulness was a product of sociability. Across discourses, there is less of a sense of cheerfulness being something that an individual cultivates inwardly, and more emphasis placed on experiencing it in a social environment. Arguably it is possible to conceive that eighteenth-century writers might have believed the power of cheerfulness was not merely psychological, but material. It might be worth considering this hypothesis alongside contemporary theories of societal interaction. How exactly immaterial things such as pleasant thoughts or polite company had tangible effects on the body was a particular area of contemporary enquiry, and one that fascinated many eighteenth-century philosophers and physicians. In the late seventeenth century, Robert Boyle had demonstrated that matter was inherently separable, transferable and shareable. For decades afterwards a big question mark hung over how exactly this might be achieved, and what the limits of such possibilities might be.[72] In the realm of natural philosophy, attention focused on how sentiments, social experiences and emotions might be shared and transferred between people. Did emotions and thoughts have a material essence that could move from person to person? Did the 'pleasurable sharing of sentiments' involve matter travelling between people like an infectious disease? What invisible powers or forces might be responsible for the sharing of psychic experiences? Various theories emerged in answer to these questions, some of which may be of relevance to the imagined operation of cheerfulness in these texts. To understand the enthusiasm with which these writers thought cheerfulness might be gleaned or stimulated by social interaction, we need to appreciate the mysterious power of social interaction in the eighteenth-century scientific imagination.

The best known of these theories of social interaction is undoubtedly 'sympathy'. Sympathy, as discussed by various eighteenth-century philosophers including Shaftesbury, Hutcheson, Hume, Smith and Kames, was essentially a framework for thinking about empathy or identification with others. It was also a key idea within the broader language of sensibility. Sympathy described an imaginative act of identification between one person and another in a social context, and was identified throughout the century as one of the binding forces in society. In the *Treatise of Human Nature* (1740), Hume suggested that sentiments could be transferred somewhat mechanically, unconsciously, and therefore experienced passively. Feelings could be almost detached from the self. Smith, in *Theory of Moral Sentiments* (1759), considered that the transmission of particles might be responsible for the transfer of sentiments between people.[73] Sympathy was but one of many ideas proffered to explain how matter might move from person to person; various theories, some infinitely more speculative than others, are mooted in eighteenth-century scientific texts. Cheyne was no stranger to the broad possibility of such concepts, having himself employed Newton's theory of the aether to argue for continuum between matter and spirit in his earlier works of natural theology. Haller thought that there was an 'electrical principle' in the air which might account for a transfer, and which, when inhaled, 'increases and diminishes by turns the alacrity of the mind'.[74] The exact nature of the invisible forces in society remained mysterious, illusive, compulsive and divisive. As Peter Otto has concluded,

> there was, of course, no agreement on the identity of these fundamental powers: magnetism, electricity, a 'most subtle spirit', a 'vitalistic fluid' and sexuality are only a few of the forces that haunt eighteenth-century medical and scientific texts.[75]

Otto's study of the fanatical James Graham, a man who managed to be both medic and magician, is but one example of the seemingly farcical limits that could be reached in imagining these mysterious forces. The self-styled 'rational mystic' and physician William Belcher and his theory of 'intellectual electricity' is another somewhat risible example. In an attempt to provide 'a practical system of the passions', Belcher claimed he had discovered that 'ELECTRICITY or OXYGEN' was 'the vehicle of Thought'.[76] Despite acknowledging that his theories would strike the reader as 'about equally posed between wisdom and folly', Belcher nonetheless 'risked' his hypothesis that human ideas were somehow conscious – or at least active and subject to the laws of matter – and able to move between people.[77] Either thoughts were 'clothed in particles of oxygenous fire' or they were 'themselves living entities and intelligences', rather like 'insects'.[78] As such, while they were 'floating in the air', they might 'strike on or enter at the eyes of persons', thereby facilitating the sharing of ideas and sentiments.[79]

A more conservative set of ideas were those inherent in the chemical science of 'pneumatology'. Pneumatology was a term of major significance throughout most of the eighteenth century. Originally a scholastic term referring to the philosophy of spirits, it became increasingly associated with the philosophy of the human spirit (psychology) and the science of the human mind as the century wore on. Pneumatic medicine focused on respiration, gases and their therapeutic powers. Interpreted broadly, pneumatology provided a number of ways of envisaging how human experience was something transferable and sharable. What was it in the air, or in the breath, that might support life; and how might the breath be a means of transferring qualities between one body and another? As Joseph Priestley acknowledged to the Royal Society in 1776, 'there is, perhaps, no subject in physiology, and very few in philosophy in general, that has engaged more attention than that of the use of respiration.'[80] The chemist and physician Thomas Beddoes (1760–1808) was among the proponents of this pneumatic medicine. He argued that social habits literally spread diseases, and his works looked forward to a conjunction between pneumatic medicine and a reformed social order. Although he focused upon the less desirable habits of snobbery, drunkenness and bad education, he also noted – as we saw earlier – that a 'cheerful temper' was an especially healthy and useful 'accomplishment' to enjoy, suggesting it might be of some considerable influence in disseminating more positive influences.[81]

The aging body was not exempt from theories of pneumatic transfer. In 1743, the German doctor Johann Heinrich Cohausen parodied chemical respiratory theory in a small but sensational book. He suggested that inhaling the breath of young women might be a means of preventing aging and facilitating long life. Although undoubtedly a farce, the book, *Hermippus Redivivus: or, The Sage's Triumph over Old Age and the Grave*, made a considerable impact at the time of its publication, went through numerous English editions and remained in print until 1847. The seemingly ludicrous theory may even have been taken perfectly seriously by some, as is suggested by the tone of the reviews in both the *Gentleman's Magazine* and the *Daily Gazeteer*.[82] The book was described as a 'Physico-Medical Dissertation', and reviewers claimed that Cohausen had 'established' a method 'on a Physical Basis' using arguments from 'Chymical Philosophy'.[83] Moreover, an unattributed synopsis of the theory was annexed to Cheyne's posthumous compendium of maxims and receipts, and even received special billing on the title page as 'An uncommon METHOD of prolonging human Life'. The popularity of the little book undoubtedly owes a great deal to the contemporary interest in health, longevity and life extension, as David Boyd-Haycock acknowledges. However, a close reading of Cohausen's cleverly argued hypothesis suggests that it is the pneumatic theories themselves that might have appeared persuasive, particularly given the contemporary interest in theories of material transfer and social interaction. Relying heavily on Boerhaave's formulation of hydraulic mechanism, Cohausen began by stating that the body was 'a pneumatico-hydraulic Machine', and that, 'with due Care' it could be 'kept in good Order'.[84] He went on to posit a radical (although not implausible) theory of pneumatic exchange between persons in social proximity:

> There seems to be nothing forced or absurd, in conceiving that the Warm, Active and Balsamic Particles thrown off by the Lungs of young People into the Air, which they Respire, may give it such a Quality, as when sucked in again by a Person in Years, shall communicate an extraordinary Force to the circulating Humours in his Body, and so quicken and enliven them, as to bestow a kind of reflective Youthfulness, which may for many Years keep off and delay those infirmities, to which People of the same Age are generally subject.[85]

Although this was a rather outlandish idea, in fact Cheyne had suggested something not dissimilar – certainly pneumatic, and via remarkably similar terminology – in one of his works published in the previous year. In *The Natural Method of Cureing the Diseases of the Body, and the Disorders of the Mind Depending on the Body* (1742), under a section entitled, 'Rules for obtaining and preserving Health in the Decline of Life', Cheyne put forward a similar suggestion. Extolling the benefits of early rising, he explained that early morning air would be 'impregnated with balsamic and fragrant Particles drawn from the lightest and sweetest Vegetables'. These, 'early-rising Persons, of a tender and delicat Frame, should strive to enjoy', whilst they were still hovering around within reach.[86] Balsamic particles in the air, whether conveyed through the breath of light, sweet girls or the emissions of light sweet vegetables might have an especial value for the aging body. What such ideas seem to suggest is that it was conceptually plausible to imagine the transfer of matter via respiration – or other more mysterious means – and that the aging body in particular might be in a position to benefit from such exchanges.

It seems plausible that eighteenth-century writers entertained notions of cheerfulness working in ways similar to these examples. At the very least it appears that medical writers referenced, or hinted at, the possibility of cheerfulness being transferred materially. Without doubt, cheerfulness could be sourced via sensory and societal stimuli. Cheerfulness appears to originate outside rather than inside the body, as in the case of Akenside's experience, and Boswell's description of cheerfulness 'breaking in'. Cheerfulness, as Addision explained, was (literally) catching:

> A cheerful Mind is not only disposed to be affable and obliging, but raises the same good Humour in those who come within its Influence. A Man finds himself well pleased, he does not know why, with the Chearfulness of his Companion: It is like a sudden Sun-shine, that awakens a secret Delight in the Mind, without her attending to it: The Heart rejoices of its own Accord, and naturally flows out into Friendship and Benevolence towards the Person who has so kindly an Effect upon it.[87]

With such thoughts in mind, one may appreciate why Samuel Richardson's house, where he held affable social and literary gatherings, was described as 'that mansion of cheerfulness and grotto of instruction'.[88] It is possible to suggest that, like sympathy, cheerfulness functioned as a binding force within society: a shared aspect of human experience. Akenside imagined that the 'Goddess' of cheerfulness, had the power to rouse 'the harmony of human souls'.[89] Buchan suggested that the mind 'took its cast' from the company around it, and from his description it seems that he may have imagined physical forces in action. In insisting that one's companions ought to be 'of sound mind', Buchan explained that a person's mental state 'diffus[ed] ... all around him, and generally taints the minds of his companions with the temper of his own'.[90] For this specific reason, it was essential that 'those who would be healthy and happy, ought therefore to associate with the young, the cheerful, and good humoured'.[91]

Perhaps the notion of 'cheerfulness' was especially apt to interpretation in these ways because of its etymological connections to things literal, consumable and shareable. For, being 'full' of 'cheer' involved the consumption of food or entertainment. 'Cheer' itself is an external, material substance that nourishes the body. Possibly it was with such thoughts in mind that Boswell described Garrick – the veritable master of entertaining provision – as 'Cheerfullest man of his age'.[92] Even if writers did not explicitly acknowledge the material, transferable potential of cheerfulness, they may at least have conveyed possibilities in the minds of their readers. When reconsidering and plagiarizing Cohausen's breath theory in his own *Valetudinarians Bath Guide: or, The Means of Obtaining Long Life and Health* (1780), Philip Thicknesse assured his readers that, 'if the breath of young people does not tend to Long Life, the society of lively cheerful people of all ages certainly does'.[93]

Conclusion

Rather like the concept of 'politeness', cheerfulness is one of those terms that appears to be quite superficial, but actually has a far deeper resonance in its eighteenth-century contexts than it does today. The similarities between cheerfulness and politeness are obvious. From a body perspective, a body under the influence of cheerfulness does seem to have a lot in common with what we have come to recognize as the 'polite' body: a body unswayed by passionate experience, socially-turned, pious, benevolent, virtuous and carefully policed. Yet more so than politeness, cheerfulness has an inherent bodily dimension, and the corporeal state that it engendered had a particular significance for the aging body. As this chapter has shown, ideas about the physical effects of cheerfulness clearly permeated more broadly than medical discourse alone. The meanings of cheerfulness expressed in periodicals, advertisements, dictionaries, poems and the like may have informed the ways that cheerfulness was discussed in the medical texts, and the nature of the advice that was consequently meted out.

Undoubtedly, cheerfulness had real power and potential in the eighteenth-century imagination. It was championed unequivocally as a force of good. It offered protection against the corruption of modern luxury-infused civilization, and the corruption represented by an ailing, failing, decaying body. Like sympathy, and other forces of society subject to extensive scrutiny in eighteenth-century natural philosophy, cheerfulness could take on the mantle of a binding force within society. Perhaps even it may be denoted a 'force of society' in its own right, and if so it deserves further investigation. Somewhat mysterious in essence, cheerfulness is an amorphous and beguiling concept: perhaps located in human nature, perhaps created through societal interaction, perhaps a material essence in itself. Yet it was an apt and useful concept for eighteenth-century writers, and one that might be harnessed to several ends: medical, social, moral and even political.

The rhetoric of cheerfulness described in this chapter represents an extension of the ideas expressed in Chapter 3, about agency over the aging body, and indeed of those about aging from the outside. In championing the power of cheerfulness over the aging body, medical writers were advocating the great potential for self-mastery and self-control; describing a body that was pliant to the will. Aging bodies were said to respond to mental discipline; not the kind that is self-serving and introverted, but that which is enjoyable and sociable, pleasant and beneficial. In emphasizing the element of choice, and in describing an aging body that responded physically to positive thinking and good company, medical writers were, on the one hand, providing quite an empowering message; one that we might not see as compatible with a Foucauldian narrative about the imposition of discipline through the medical establishment. On the other hand, by endorsing a very particular type of outlook and behaviour – above all one of calmness, restraint and mental levity – medical writers were indeed shaping the parameters of acceptable sociable conduct. This is the subject of the following chapter.

5 AGED IDENTITIES: PRESCRIPTIVE BEHAVIOUR FOR 'OLD MEN'

Introduction

This chapter considers the representation of 'aged identity' in medical advice literature. I extract from these books a sense of how eighteenth-century doctors could shape reader's behaviours, actions and aspirations; reaching beyond their remit as purely medical guides and becoming disseminators of prescriptive self-fashioning in old age. Here we examine medical advice as an important platform for the delivery of normalized identity in 'polite' society: part of the burgeoning eighteenth-century literature of conduct. The previous chapter established just how important cheerfulness and sociability were for the management of aging. I suggest here that it is precisely because eighteenth-century doctors were so concerned with psychosomatic and social cures that it is possible to investigate medical texts for ideas about conduct, self-fashioning and identity. They show us some of the idealized representations of old age extant at this time and what the medical cadre defined as acceptable behaviour for older people. In essence, we can detect here a particular representation of eighteenth-century 'aged identity' – if I may call it that.

The very first point to note is that mining medical advice literature for representations of aged identities does not present us with a variety of representations, but one very specific formulation. This formulation is also exclusive, for medical advice addresses not old *people* but old *men*. Hence it is this unique representation of aged identity that this chapter will present: the often eponymous 'old man' of medical advice. In order to contextualize this figure, I juxtapose him against other 'identities' on offer in eighteenth-century England, particularly the hegemonic form of masculinity extant in this period: the 'polite gentleman' identified by the historiography. Hence, this chapter also contributes to the history of masculinity in eighteenth-century England, and in fact it fills something of a gap in the historiography of that subject. As I am at pains to point out, scholars in this field have been largely unaware of how age and aging affects constructions of masculinity. Although there have been several studies that investigate the various masculinities existing in eighteenth-century England, few of them have paid any attention to the old or aging man. Finally, although my conclusions pertain largely to the historiography of aging, masculinity and of polite society, I do nudge my findings onto a broader historiographical stage. Although it is impossible to draw solid conclusions about gender from a study that focuses on men, I close by offering some tentative suggestions around some of the grand narratives that characterize the historiography of the eighteenth century, proposing that the introduction of age and aging into eighteenth-century gender studies may provide some important challenges to the historiography of 'modernization'.

Old Men as Readers and Writers

Regardless of whether we choose to interpret Enlightenment interest in combating aging and extending life as an overtly male endeavour, the market for medical advice literature was certainly not exclusively for men. G. S. Rousseau lists a number of eighteenth-century advice books concerned with health and bodily management aimed exclusively at women.[1] The market for medical advice certainly overlapped with that of writings of a broadly 'sensible' nature, of which women were certainly avid readers. Cheyne referred to his readers as 'persons' rather than 'men', and we know that many of his followers were women. It was possible for writers to use the word 'man' in a default, generic human sense without having to gender their advice or readers. Yet despite the above considerations, it is still a simple fact that it is old men rather than old women who are assumed to be readers in these books, and it is old men rather than old women imagined in illustrative examples. There are, I suggest, particular reasons for this near exclusively male focus.

Firstly, as medical advice became more concerned with psychosomatism and sociability, there was greater formal need to imagine a subject. Although mental stability had always been considered important in old age, advice now abounded with statements of a 'psychological' nature. 'Nothing, in a man's life', wrote Dr Trusler, 'tends more to health and longevity, than peace of mind; it is the index to old age.'[2] The novel consequence of this was that authors often imagined a protagonist – an 'old man' – in a societal context and with an individual identity. Also, as a result of this psychological turn, some writers – especially Cheyne – began to talk to their readers specifically about how to conduct themselves, especially in society. John Hill opened his *Old Man's Guide to Health and Longer Life* of 1750 with the bold statement that it was his purpose to ensure the 'antient' knew how to 'conduct themselves' in social situations.[3] Advice given by Fothergill – a habitual correspondent in the *Gentleman's Magazine* – focused as much on the presentation of the aged self *to others* as the inward, individual health of the body. 'Men in years', he advised, should 'be assiduous in keeping their bodies clean and neat ... their minds contented and cheerful, and render their behaviour and conversation agreeable.'[4] When introducing his *Comforts of Old Age* in 1816, Sir Thomas Bernard insisted that his advice was written in 'the interest of our friends, connections, and dependants' and 'the welfare of the community'.[5] His chapters treated of 'social intercourse', 'self-examination' and 'melioration of temper': a true self-fashioning for old age, with a close eye on the perception of the old man and the identity he might present.

Secondly, medical advice became unashamedly more personal and autobiographical. Many authors identified themselves openly as old men, even boasted of their longevity. Cheyne published the autobiography of his 'own crazy Carcase', telling the story of how despite hedonistic binges in early life (he expanded to thirty-two stones in weight), consequent reform and regimen ensured that he enjoyed 'as good Health, as, at my Time of Life (being now *Sixty*), I, or any Man, can reasonably expect'.[6] The doctor introduced a friendly, conversational, *ad hominem* approach. Always 'begging the Pardon of the Reader' for 'troubling him' with 'private Matters', he sympathized with, identified with and motivated his readers, creating a platform for self-conscious self-representation as old or ailing men. Trusler, whose oeuvre included numerous conduct works like *Principles of Politeness*, advertised his *Sure Way to Strengthen Life with Vigour, particularly in Old Age* (1770) as being written at the age of eighty-four, 'without spectacles' and 'with a full possession of mental powers'. In a conversational preface he congratulated himself on not writing 'like a physician', but rather as one who wished to share with 'every man of common understanding' his personal experiences of old age.[7] Similarly, the anonymous author of *The Invalid* (1804) offered reflections on 'self management' from 'the experience and example of one who ... is arrived on the verge of ninety years'.[8] As an upshot of the advice becoming increasingly more autobiographical, sociable and 'polite', it also became more specifically about old *men*, constituting as it did an imagined dialogue between old male writers and old male readers. It is aged masculinity (rather than femininity) therefore, that we are presented with in these texts.

Eighteenth-Century Masculinities

In the last twenty years, a number of studies have sought to uncover what – in theory if not always in practice – it meant to be 'masculine' in eighteenth-century England. Although it was never the case that there was one simple set of rules for all men in all situations, scholarship confirms that there was a 'hegemonic' form of idealized masculinity: polite gentlemanliness.[9] In contrast to early modern 'manhood' characterized by patriarchy and honour, and distinct also from Victorian 'manliness' (which has been identified with etiquette, taciturnity and domesticity), eighteenth-century masculinity was first and foremost defined by 'politeness'.[10] First described by Paul Langford and Lawrence Klein, 'polite' society emerged as a consequence of late seventeenth-century socio-economic change and the political settlement surrounding the Glorious Revolution. At the dawn of the eighteenth century, the nation was seen to be more powerful, prosperous, tolerant and civilized, and the concept of politeness functioned as a 'master metaphor' to indicate the newly desirable qualities of civility, good breeding, manners, easiness and gentility.[11] As Philip Carter explains, politeness became 'the means to acquire a suitably refined, yet virtuous' masculinity that appeared 'both novel and superior to existing forms of manly virtue'.[12] Now, being masculine meant being mannered, urbane, civilized, and perhaps most importantly, knowing to behave and converse in company with a requisite amount of self-restraint, rendering oneself pleasant and agreeable in the process. Manners in particular became instrumental in the demonstration of polite gentlemanliness: they were, as Anthony Fletcher explains, 'the centrepiece' of polite society.[13] It was this 'complete system of manners and conduct based on the arts of conversation' that was set down in a wealth of conduct literature, periodicals and self-help manuals for self-fashioning men of artisan class and above.[14]

However, polite gentlemanliness was neither unproblematic nor ubiquitous. It was, according to Michèle Cohen, 'rent with anxieties, in particular the anxiety about effeminacy'.[15] Critics were also troubled by the potential inauthenticity that could be concealed by overly mannered conduct. Recent studies have drawn attention to the fact that there were alternative masculinities on offer besides the hegemonic ideal. 'The fop, the libertine, the homosexual, the religious man … the pretty man and blackguard … the reader of erotica and the violent aggressor', write Tim Hitchcock and Michèle Cohen, were all 'possible male identities' that could be occupied in this period.[16] Most recently Matthew McCormack has shown how political identity – especially the notion of 'independence', connoting autonomy, self-mastery, conscience and individual responsibility – contributed to constructions of masculinity in Georgian England.[17] In sum, although scholarship has been notably lighter in determining whether represented ideal types were reflected in practice, we do now have a clear grasp of the distinctive ideas eighteenth-century readers might encounter about their society's conception of masculinity.

However, what is glaringly absent from these studies – at least to one used to working on aging – is the figure of the old or aging man, and the masculinity to which he might aspire. In marked contrast to the work done on masculinity in the sixteenth and seventeenth centuries, the age criterion is either missing entirely from scholarship on eighteenth-century masculinity, or historians focus upon the transition from youth to full adult maturity.[18] This may be partly explained by the source material favoured: conduct books often describe an abstracted ideal type, forever in stasis in time and space. The idealized polite gentleman is often presumed antecedently to be of certain means, education and political rights. To this list of unspoken perquisites we might add that he is also presumed not to be an old or aging man. Also, many conduct books followed the established format of 'father-son' advice, and hence were aimed specifically at young men making an entrance into the world of psychological independence. Whereas it has been acknowledged that young men required instruction in order to make themselves truly masculine, there has been no parallel consideration of how an aging man might be instructed to confirm or redefine his masculinity in the later stages of life. Hence, historians have tended to treat masculinity as a static form of identity, with little regard to the inescapable fact that like all forms of personal identity, masculinities are made and remade over life and time.

The historiography seems to suggest that the concept of masculinity was in fact becoming more inclusive in this period. Scholars have noted a terminological shift from early modern discussions of 'manhood' to eighteenth-century considerations of 'masculinity'.[19] Not merely an etymological issue, this marks a significant epistemological shift. In the sixteenth and seventeenth centuries, as Alexandra Shepard explains, the concept of 'manhood' denoted a particular stage in the life cycle and was defined negatively against 'youth' and 'old age'.[20] Limited to a mere ten or twenty years, manhood could be understood as a temporal category: one from which old men were necessarily excluded. By contrast, 'masculinity' in its eighteenth-century guise was a concept closer to our own understandings of the word: a set of abstract characteristics, technically open to all and more a matter for the individual conscience.

Representations of Old Age

The aged masculinity that we are about to discover was but one representation of aged identity that polite readers might have encountered. Certain prescriptive images of old age and of aged masculinity were extant; both the Biblical and Classical traditions offered well-established depictions. The twelfth chapter of *Ecclesiastes* civilly compared the decline of life to the close of the season and provided the basis for the idea that old age should be a time of quiet acceptance, retirement, self-examination, piety and preparation for death. Cicero's *De Senectute* was popular in translation throughout the century and formed the basis for Bernard's *Comforts of Old Age*.[21] Describing the potential for a wise, contemplative old age, the work provided the basic template for the grey-bearded venerable patriarch or magistrate. Other depictions described old age as pitiful, hateful and painful. Late seventeenth-century moralizers such as the Dissenting Minister Richard Steele – whose *Discourse on Old Age* was reprinted throughout the eighteenth century – saw old age as a time when one came closer to God, but also as harbinger of avarice, selfishness and fear. Roger Bacon's *Cure of Old Age and*

Preservation of Youth, originally written in the thirteenth century but translated and paraphrased in the eighteenth, was another frequent frame of reference. Bacon described old age as a disease with repugnant physical manifestations such as 'filthy spitting' and 'rotten Phlegm'.[22] In reality too, as Susannah Ottaway confirms, the eighteenth century was 'no golden age of aging', and work by Pat Thane and Lynn Botelho confirms the harsh realities attendant on a declining body, especially for the poor.

The Cheerful Old Man of Medical Advice

If the ideal eighteenth-century gentleman was first and foremost 'polite', his older counterpart in medical advice was ideally 'cheerful'. As the previous chapter demonstrated, cheerfulness was *the* aspirational quality to be striven for in old age, and references to cheerfulness (as opposed to any other arbitrarily chosen synonym) abound in medical advice, often coupled with – but never surpassed by – other epithets such as 'ease', 'serenity' or 'tranquillity'. Cheerfulness had much in common with politeness, especially its emphasis on sociability and its opposition to introversion. Although cheerfulness had been a recognized route to longevity since Aristotle, it was in the eighteenth century that it became identified as a desirable *sociable* quality in old age and, we might say, a particular code of aged masculinity. By advocating cheerful behaviours, medical writers could connect proscribed therapeutic behaviour in old age to codes of polite behaviour, linking polite gentlemanliness and aged masculinity. However, the cheerful old man was no carbon copy of the polite gentleman, for cheerfulness carried certain associations that medical writers were only too keen to emphasize in order to keep the two distinct.

As Philip Carter explains, eighteenth-century gentlemanly masculinity was predominantly 'a sociable category' in which gender identity was conferred by man's capacity for 'gentlemanly social performance'.[23] Like the polite gentleman, the old man was rendered cheerful by his interactions with others, particularly via the medium of conversation. Doctors insisted that the old man make his conversation light, easy and entertaining, both to moderate his own subcutaneous functions and, importantly, to make himself presentable and affable to others. Cheyne suggested dispelling the 'Damps' of old age with 'warm Fires and cheerful Conversation' surrounded by 'healthy' servants, children and bedfellows.[24] 'Nothing will more effectually contribute towards the Felicity of a *Green Old Age*', he insisted, 'than innocent and entertaining *Amusements*, engageing and light Studies, and rational *Diversions in* cheerful and affectionat Society'.[25] Certain lighter wines were recommended specifically because they afforded 'more Room for long *Conversation* and Chearfulness', and reading material should 'supply the mind with cheerful and pleasing ideas' to 'furnish conversation in society'.[26]

Authors even prioritized sociable behaviours over strict temperance or dietetic regimen. Although everyone agreed it was important to be moderate in old age, this should not be observed too rigorously as to hamper social fluidity. Following his various recommendations for temperance in eating, the anonymous author of *The Invalid* insisted that if an old man were to find himself 'present at a festival entertainment', he should 'enter freely into the humour of the company' and 'be as *merry* as the best of them'. 'Nay stand upon your head and drink a bumper to the Antipodes ... if that be the taste of the company', he enthused. Although not technically desirable, this was infinitely preferable to pedantic, introverted abstention. 'Nothing' was 'more disgusting or unpolite' than an old man who prioritized a 'selfish' regard to his own health'.[27] Bernard agreed. In old age it was especially pertinent to 'disincumber the mind of all selfish and irritable feelings' and to cherish 'gentle and conciliating manners'.[28] Like the codifiers of gentlemanly conduct, physicians understood that both health and identity in old age needed to be achieved outwardly – cheerfulness was a sociable category.

It was especially important for old men to mix with young company. Those celebrating instances of longevity often drew attention to the fact that the epic hero of abstemious regimen, the fifteenth-century Venetian Luigi Cornaro, was forever in the company of his many grandchildren in his last years. Philip Thicknesse thought there no 'better sign of Long Life in old men' than 'their being of a lively, sociable disposition, and fond of young company'. Frenchmen, he thought, deserved to be celebrated in this respect: their longevity might be attributed to the fact that they never gave up 'the society of young women, nor any young company', till they were 'unable to keep any'.[29] When the German doctor Christoph Hufeland set about determining the principles of longevity in 1794, he determined 'the frame of mind best fitted and most beneficial to old age', was that produced by 'intercourse with children and young people'. As he explained, 'their innocent pastime and youthful frolics have something which tend, as it were, to renovate and revive'.[30] In order to promote 'cheerfulness and suavity of manners' Bernard advised trying to 'assimilate' ones manners to those of the young. It made one so much more presentable. As his aged protagonist explained, 'I find ... that they listen with much more pleasure and attention to any advice.'[31] William Buchan apparently put such recommendations into practice. If his obituarist is to be believed, the doctor owed much of his cheerfulness in later life to his preference 'for the society of the young'. For 'in order to enjoy it' he apparently 'fixed his residence near the Chapter Coffee-House' during the last years of his life.[32]

It might be worth making a brief digression into the coffee house here. Understood as the epitome of the public sphere, the coffee house has attracted a good deal of scholarly attention, not least concerning the issue of whether they were exclusively homosocial. That Buchan's obituarist saw them as characteristic of youth might invite other questions about the *age* as well as the sex of the clientele. For our purposes however, the assumption that such places would not usually be occupied by the old might suggest that the potential for intergenerational interaction was quite limited outside the family or domestic sphere. Writers of medical advice – in advocating close interaction with the young – may have been recommending a practice that was ambitious in its deviation from cultural norms. We know little in fact about intergenerational sociability in eighteenth-century culture, as studies of theatres, coffee houses, masquerades and pleasure gardens have been more concerned with the interactions between those of different sex and social standing.

Another aspect of this cheerful behavioural code for old and aging men was that it was contrasted against excess and luxury, and was characterized by moderation. Here cheerfulness mirrored politeness, for the stigmatization of excess one of the core tenets of polite society. The notion of excess and its 'connotations of luxury and self-indulgence', Michèle Cohen explains, 'positioned the gentleman as effeminate, whereas 'self-control positioned him as manly'.[33] Cheerfulness was sedate and sober, and did not involve effusive displays of mirth. Within medical advice, the word 'cheerful' functioned as a stamp of approval for habits, pursuits and behaviours characterized by moderation and sociability. In suggesting that the 'old man' be 'always cheerful but never merry', Hill recommended an hour or two of conversation with family or neighbours before retiring early to bed.[34]

Just as the 'polite gentleman' of conduct literature had an unwelcome alter-ego – the effeminate man with his 'Frenchified' manners – the cheerful old man of medical advice had his own anti-hero: the pedantic, introverted aging scholar.[35] Although the tension between scholarship and sociability was 'much discussed' in the eighteenth century, the fact that 'the life of the mind left men in danger of becoming dull and anti-social' was a point that needed particular emphasis in old age.[36] A contrite Cheyne condemned his own 'vanity' in pursuing 'airy studies', describing them as 'pernicious to society'.[37] Writers unified in their insistence that a 'scholarly' old man was both necessarily unhealthy and socially unwelcome. Doctors often cautioned that 'intense thinking' wore out the constitution 'more than the most laborious exercise', and agreed that it was the mind 'naturally inclined to moderation in its exertions' that was most healthful and appropriate for old age.[38] As we saw previously, cheerfulness was juxtaposed not only against 'sadness', but also against 'profound thought' and 'a degree of thoughtlessness' recommended as 'necessary' for longevity.[39] Hufeland went further, suggesting that introverted scholarship was best demeaned as a kind of luxury. He defined mental exertion in exactly these terms, setting out to clarify 'what is to be understood by debauchery or excess in the function of thinking'.[40] The cheerful old man did not retreat into his study or allow himself to be consumed by abstruse or selfish thought. For some writers, a certain levity was considered aspirational. A point on which everyone agreed was that the stereotype most likely to achieve longevity was the witless country bumpkin – largely on account of how little he taxed his mental powers.

The ideal of restricted mental expenditure was quite a counterpoint to the image of the learned Ciceronian patriarch. This is not to say that medical advice opposed explicitly the Ciceronian ideal or rendered it any less *venerable*, but that views about the physical toll of mental exertion – now explicable in neural terms – did offer a challenge to the established idea of a philosophical old age on *health* grounds. It also – again implicitly – offered a gentle challenge to the traditional Biblical view of old age as a period of inner reflection. Sermon literature drawing upon Ecclesiastes tended to emphasize meditation and self-examination as the correct activities for the old, whereas without specifically advising against spiritual activities of this nature, medical writers coaxed their readers away from introspection and into cosy domesticity or wider society. However, it should be emphasized that there was nothing exclusively secular about the cheerful old man and his sociability. Although cheerfulness led to secular pursuits, its origin was a keen sense of piety and duty. As the devout Cheyne, whose work was always underpinned by a heavily spiritual agenda, was careful to keep reminding his readers, 'the *Love of God*' was 'the most *powerful* of all the *Means* of *Health* and *Long Life*'.[41] Although the degree of overt devotion in his works was unusual for writings in the medical genre, the connection between cheerfulness and a fatalistic acceptance of the divine plan and His benevolence was never far away.

In many ways then, the idealized cheerful old man of medical literature was an extension of the polite gentleman: a calm sociable conversationalist whose health and sense of self depended on his interaction with those around him. Yet in one important way, cheerfulness actually distanced the old man from his younger counterpart. Sexuality played no part in the construction of aged masculinity. Although it is acknowledged that eighteenth-century understandings of hegemonic masculinity were more concerned with the *social* rather than the *sexual* aspects of male behaviour, this did not entail a wholesale dismissal of the polite gentleman's active (hetero)sexuality. As John Barrell explains, it became 'important to invent narratives of civic emancipation from sexuality' because 'manly virtue' was seen to be 'effeminized by submission to female charms'.[42] Emancipation from sexual desire stood as a mark of masculinity, but this narrative inherently confirmed rather than denied the presence of the gentlemanly libido. By contrast, there was a committed – and often disgusted – drive to distance the old man from his sexual past.

Once past the 'meridian of life', both male and female bodies, Cheyne thought, became somewhat sexless. Indeed, his vision of the aged body was akin to what has become known as the 'one-sex' model. The 'Difference of the *Sexes*' was to be found only in 'the different *Configuration* of the superinduc'd Crust or Shell laid over the primitive *aetherial* Body', which was, he thought 'pretty near of the same Figure, Size and Materials, originally'.[43] Although the female 'climacteric' (menopause) was the more visibly obvious, the change happened 'equally to both the *Sexes*', 'a *general Law* of *Nature*'. Furthermore, Cheyne not only posited a 'natural' end to sexuality, but also managed to equate this exit from sexuality with an exit from full adulthood. Old age was a mere 'dotage and childhood'.[44] Old men had to 'be treated, and treat themselves', he cautioned, 'much in the same way as a Child must be treated in his *Non-age*, till he arrives at Manhood'.[45] In ceasing to be virile, one ceased to be adult, and returned to the genderless status occupied by children. For Cheyne then, old age was both distinct physiologically from manhood and comparable to infancy. To put this in modern terms, we might say that gender was, in Cheyne's eyes, a thoroughly adult identity that ended at a certain biological point.

Comparisons between old age and infancy were common throughout the century, and old age was frequently referred to as a second childhood. Although Hill thought it 'only in the extreme of age that men become children again', nonetheless the physical proximity of old age and infancy he could not deny: 'weakness is weakness whether it be in old men or children'.[46] Any attempts at expressions of virility at this stage of life were futile because unnatural. Should sexual indulgence take place, the old man would soon be, as Fothergill put it, 'demolished'.[47] By 1836, James Johnson was denying that 'second childishness and mere oblivion' would overcome men by the age of seventy.[48] But his objection was based on Shakespeare's allegorical timing of the event rather than its eventual inevitability. Despite not calling old age a second childhood, Johnson thought the seventh decade a time defined by the paucity of basic need and the absence of sexual desire. 'In this late stage of the journey, our wants, and even our wishes are few, and easily satisfied.'[49]

Those who portrayed life as a spiritual journey could tell a similar story in different terms. Bernard's definition of 'cheerfulness' as the ultimate aspiration for old men was heavily imbued with a Ciceronian sense of spiritual 'progress from sensual to intellectual enjoyment', where through 'instruction, experience and example' the '*animal*' would be converted into a '*rational*' being.[50] When quizzed about '*sexual* Passion', Bernard's nonagenarian protagonist replied that 'connubial love' would inevitably 'refine and become intellectual' or 'spiritual'.[51] Ultimately, cheerfulness was a means of denying aged sexuality: a state that signalled both freedom and distance from the passions and desires that defined earlier stages of a man's life.

That aged sexuality was reviled universally is obvious from the mass of popular printed material about 'May and December' marriages: those partnerships of great disparity in age examined in Chapter 2. The subject was a well established and enduring topic of poems, plays, jokes and ballads, and the stereotypes of youth and age were well-worn characters. Not surprisingly, Karen Harvey confirms that old male bodies were treated extremely 'harshly' in eighteenth-century erotica, and any attempts 'to enhance the potency of older men' portrayed as 'desperate'.[52] There was, however, a significant eighteenth-century exception to this trend. Beginning in the 1740s, Cohausen's rejuvenation theory drew considerable attention in the medical and the polite world, and it rested on being able to imagine the positive benefits an aging male body might gain from associating with a young female one. The theory that old men might be rejuvenated by inhaling the breath of healthy young women was an ancient one, but although the Classical theory was premised on the breath of youth rather than the breath of young women per se, it was the old man / young woman relationship that was exploited in the eighteenth century. This was sensational satire, with sexy overtones. Both Cohausen and his English translator commented extensively on the possibility of creating a 'college' of nubile young virgins to generate a supply of 'balsamic breaths', and Cohausen even went as far as suggesting the benefits could be taken to a 'higher pitch' if old men 'lay with' the breathy girls. In 1780, Philip Thicknesse imagined a modern-day equivalent in contemporary Bath, a place without equal when it came to making up the 'prescription' with 'so lovely of the sex', he thought. Setting himself up as an old man with a keen sense of sensual, if not sexual, enjoyment, he boasted thus to his readers: 'I am myself turned sixty ... yet, having always partaken of the breath of young women whenever they lay in my way, I feel none of those infirmities which so often strike my eyes and ears in this great city.'[53] However, Thicknesse was keen to keep away from overtly carnal suggestions. Should his readers wish to put theory into practice, they would be merely 'innocently indulging themselves in one of the most pleasing gratifications that the human *mind* can enjoy'.[54] Careful not to cast himself as a lecherous sallier, he finally tempered with a more conservative remark echoing received opinion: 'If the breath of young people does not tend to Long Life, the society of lively cheerful people of all ages certainly does.'[55]

It seems that cheerfulness was most applicable to and achievable for *aging* rather than very old men. Although writers sometimes claimed to be in their eighties and nineties, the cheerful old man of medical advice was most likely not decrepit. Most authors presumed their readers had a certain ability to exercise, to socialize, to hear well enough to partake in conversations, see well enough to read novels, even perhaps ogle young women. It is clear that the cheerful old man still held onto a degree of 'independence' (that key aspect of Georgian masculinity identified by Matthew McCormack) and that he had not been reduced to the level of 'effeminate' or emasculating 'dependency'.[56] Hence the old man might not be able to retain his 'cheerful' identity right up until death's door. Cheerfulness was also socially exclusive. It obviously required a certain degree of comfort: a leisured family to read to; a social circuit; without doubt a retired lifestyle without manual labour. Books often directed old men to move away from cities, presuming there would be adequate funds to acquire an alternative, perhaps additional, country seat. Some texts presupposed a certain level of education or familiarity with improving texts. In this sense, cheerfulness aligns with politeness as something that might be aspired to by artisan classes and above, but that was rendered easier and perhaps more 'manly' by its being attended with comfort and security.

Whether in reality old men sought to live a life of cheerfulness is a question beyond the remit of this chapter, focussing as it does on ideals, prescriptions and representations. Although health and longevity guides were undoubtedly popular, we know little about whether the advice was applied. Autobiographical comments and authorial prefaces should not, however be discounted as (albeit limited) examples of theory in practice. We have already seen how Buchan apparently sought out society in the Chapter Coffee-House. Cheyne himself managed to live the life of aged cheerfulness, although with a strictness and devotion that must have been beyond the patience of many. A stickler for dietetic medicine, part of being 'lightsome and cheerful', for Cheyne, was to commit to a punishing diet. In his later years he was eating milk and biscuits only, weighed out to obsessive proportions. With this kind of role model, some readers must surely have agreed with the pronouncements of Philip Thicknesse. As he told his readers: 'Dr. Cheney and many other ingenious men have wrote on this important subject, but all of them have laid down such rigid rules of abstemiousness, that few men have resolution enough to pursue the means.'[57] The continued interest in Cohausen's breath rejuvenation theory – it went through numerous editions and languages and stayed in print until 1847 – is perhaps testament to the appeal of the alternative.

Conclusion

In describing the cheerful old man I have shown how politeness – that 'key eighteenth century paradigm' – shaped prescribed conduct for men in old age as it did in earlier life. This is not surprising given that both conduct books and medical literature shared a common language of nervous sensitivity, sensibility and sociability. However, although echoing the definitive themes of polite gentlemanliness, the cheerful old man of medical advice was distanced from his younger counterpart through a denial of his sexual identity. Hence, although aspects of polite gentlemanliness could be extended – cheerfully – to aging men, aging could be represented as a process that served to deny rather than confirm maleness or masculinity. Despite the many masculinities that adult men could occupy in this period then, it seems that old age may still have been conceptually quite different from 'masculinity' itself.

In medical literature, cheerfulness was a behavioural code prescribed for old men and demonstrated by the figure of the 'old man'. But was cheerfulness itself an exclusively male code? Writers were clear that there was a definite way to regulate, comport and present oneself in old age, and this could replicate many of the essentials of polite gentlemanliness. However, more emphasis seems to have fallen upon the importance of asserting *politeness* and *gentleness* rather than *manliness* per se. Indeed, adjectives like 'manly' or 'masculine' occur rarely in these texts. Certain forms of exercise – riding especially – could be given the epithet 'manly'.[58] Billiards, as Cheyne wrote to Samuel Richardson in a correspondence kept up in their old age, was a 'charming and manly diversion'.[59] Yet further assertions of masculinity are notably absent: masculinity itself was not something that needed to be asserted or defended. The 'old man' was not defined negatively against an old woman and the anti-hero of the piece was not threatened by 'effeminacy' but by his propensity to be short-lived or bore in company.

Some of the attributes of the cheerful old man might be equally applicable to old women. There is no reason to suggest that domestic felicity, polite conversation, piety, light reading (which might extend to novels), gentle exercise like walking, or spending time with young people would be wholly inappropriate for the polite older woman. It would also be presumptuous to suggest that the mental fortitude and self-discipline envisaged for the attainment of the psychosomatic calmness was an exclusively male preserve. Certainly Anne Kugler's study of Lady Sarah Cowper confirms that this learned, aging gentlewoman set out to create an identity based on sober piety and a keen sense of the impropriety of anything even verging on sexualized or showy behaviour.[60] Hence, although it has been possible to extract a code of aged masculinity from these texts, it does not necessarily follow that this code applied exclusively to men. Put differently, although this code was articulated through the figure of the 'old man', the 'old man' was not heavily gendered.

I want briefly to speculate about the relative importance of masculinity – indeed sex and gender *tout court* – to ideas about aging and old age in eighteenth-century England. Crudely summarized, the long eighteenth century is typically seen to witness the '*ontologizing via embodiment*' of human experience and identity.[61] It is the period said to have given birth to modern notions of gender based on notions of binary sexual difference and rooted in a modern, internalized sense of self. Medical advice in particular is typically seen as instrumental in bringing about new gender roles. What we might expect, therefore, are findings that suggest advice about aging was becoming increasingly gendered.

Yet it must be acknowledged that this does not appear to be the case. Most eighteenth-century texts on aging, health and longevity are not actually concerned with issues of sex or gender at all. Rarely did books make distinctions between male and female aging. If we look beyond texts providing medical advice for laymen to the theories of the medical establishment this is equally the case. The century's strictest physiological texts that are seen to provide the most 'scientific' descriptions of aging – Hermann Boerhaave's *Institutions in Physick* and Albrecht von Haller's *First Lines of Physiology* – continued to present an aging body without gender. Nor did authors of English medical advice identify their readers predominantly by sex. Distinctions of rank were more likely, and later texts, for example Sinclair's *Code of Health and Longevity* (1807), identified their target audience by profession. As we might expect, the exception was when fertility was the issue, but as we have seen from Cheyne's discussion, this could be used to collapse rather than affirm difference of sex. After the climacteric, sex ceased to be important.

Although it is impossible to be definitive without further research, it is worth reflecting on why aging might not have been subject to the same biologizing, medicalizing forces that are said to have created modern concepts of sex and gender during the period. For one thing, the eighteenth-century idea of aging continued to take into account many different forces – spiritual, cosmological, even astrological – and not just the secular or 'biological' issues that might be subject to paradigm shifts in physiology. As Susannah Ottaway confirms, throughout the eighteenth century, the life cycle continued to be the predominant way of conceptualizing life. Also, the overweening presence of the body spiritual continued to pervade the most authoritative and the most popular writings on the aging body. It was not simply that the health conscious old man should strive to be – in the words of Jeremy Gregory – *homo religiosus*, but that aging itself was not yet a secularized issue. Searching broadly across genres for eighteenth-century works on aging confirms the subject was as likely to be the preserve of ministers as it was medics.[62] In essence, the very idea of aging in the eighteenth-century imagination was stubbornly pre-modern and not yet ripe for medicalization or modernization in the way that gender may have been.

To come full circle, I began by noting how eighteenth-century historians have largely ignored the age factor when investigating masculine identity. In fact in the historical discipline as a whole we have been too ready to treat aspects of identity as being rather static. Despite the volume of work on identity, relatively little attention has been paid to considering how identities change over the life course. Although a category of identity in its own right, age intersects with and affects other categories of identity, especially gender. Age draws attention to the inherent instability of identity concepts, and – in the case of this study – has shown that masculinities like all identities are not about permanence, but constantly under construction.

6 IDENTITY FORMATIONS: AGE AND 'CHARACTER'

Introduction

Defining exactly what was meant by a 'person' in an eighteenth-century context has fascinated historians and philosophers alike, and has spawned an impressive historiography.[1] The same conundrum was fascinating for our eighteenth-century forebears. As Felicity Nussbaum explains, 'in eighteenth century England, "identity", "self", "soul" and "person" were dangerous and disputed formations' that spawned 'heated rhetorical battles ... about the mystery of human identity'.[2] This chapter explores this mystery from one particular angle – an age perspective – and considers a few specific and previously unexplored questions: How did eighteenth-century writers conceive age to affect the notion of the 'person' and the 'character' of that person? Did changes in character that occurred throughout life and the life cycle mean that people were said to experience multiple identities throughout life? Were these sorts of changes inherently destabilizing to the unit of the individual? By asking these questions, we engage with a key historical debate about formations of identity in eighteenth-century England – the rise of the individual agent, or making of the modern 'self'. Using age as a lens for investigating the nature of personhood, I argue, challenges the hegemonic historical narrative and draws attention to alternative identity formations still alive in the eighteenth-century imagination.

By using age as a heuristic device, we draw attention to two particular aspects of personhood that scholars have been prone to overlook: the body-centric aspect and the longitudinal, changeable aspect. Nowadays we tend to want to locate personhood and character in mental activity, above the physical caprice of the body. Yet eighteenth-century notions of personhood, as this chapter will demonstrate, continued to be very dependent on the physical self: on configurations flesh and blood. In the eighteenth century, the terms 'person' and 'character' had physiological meanings quite distinct from the kind of mental conundrums that we associate with them today. Furthermore, they were not stable concepts, but inherently referenced notions of change, time, temperament and life cycle: the ideas we encountered in Chapter 2. I want to show that written into eighteenth-century concepts of personhood were ideas about the aging, changing body; a capacity for a fluid, dynamic identity which took its value from the protean, diachronic potential of the body and the changes it experienced through the life course.

The Story of the Self

Before progressing, it is wise to be clear about terminology, especially since the accepted historiography relies heavily on semantics. In this chapter, 'personhood' refers simply to the unit of the individual: a person is one distinct psychosomatic entity. The term 'identity' is considered here to be something of an umbrella concept. It incorporates all the various possible aspects that help construct a person's sense of who they are, collectively or individually: character, body, race, class, gender and age. 'Identity' then, refers to the various concepts on offer that may help a person make sense of themselves: a set of ideas that may be drawn upon for definition. Implicitly, it also represents the inherent potential for historical difference: recognition that eighteenth-century identity concepts were a different set of ideas to our own. By contrast, the term 'self' has a very specific meaning in this chapter, and one in keeping with the accepted historiography. Here it might be wise to appropriate the definition provided by Dror Wahrman in his controversial study of identity in eighteenth-century England. 'The self', Wahrman explains,

> stands for a very particular understanding of personal identity, one that presupposes an essential core of selfhood characterized by psychological depth, or interiority, which is the bedrock of unique, expressive individual identity.[3]

The term 'self' has come to represent modernity. It represents a current, Western emphasis on the personal, interior and immaterial aspects of personhood. The 'self' is the current definition of what being a person involves in twenty-first century, one 'that embodies and bolsters core Western values' of 'authenticity and individuality'.[4] Also implicit in the term 'self' is the notion of rationality, consciousness and free will. As Charles Taylor explains, 'philosophers consider that to be a person in the full sense you have to be an agent with a sense of yourself as an agent'.[5] Historians and philosophers have laboured considerably in explaining how and when we came to inhabit this particular notion of our 'selves' as characterized by interiority, depth, individuality and agency. It is to the story of the self that we now turn.

The first scholar to state explicitly that other societies, including those in the past, had different identity concepts was the sociologist Marcel Mauss.[6] Rather than 'existing as the primordial innate idea, clearly engraved since Adam in the innermost depths of our being', Mauss argued that notions of personal identity are created by contingent worldviews: social, cultural, legal and political.[7] In a seminal essay of 1938, he described identity concepts as 'categories of the human mind'. Before we came to understand our selves as 'selves', we configured personhood very differently, Mauss explained. In explaining how this came about, Mauss essentially created a progression narrative. He told a story of how relatively primitive notions of the person developed into our modern notion of interior, conscious, psychic 'selves'.[8] His essay provided 'a summary catalogue' of different 'forms' of identity that had existed in other societies, according to their various 'systems of law, religion, customs, social structures and mentality'.[9] In Mauss' narrative, the first and most primitive identity concept was the 'character', 'role', or 'persona'. This was, he explained, a superficial, or theatrical notion of the person. For like the role assumed by an actor, the persona was located in rights, duties, titles, names and even masks or body paint, and bore no relation to any sense of an inner conscience.[10] Then, in ancient Rome, the notion of the 'persona' was given supplementary significance as the locus of legal rights and citizenship: this formulation Mauss called the 'person'.[11] Notions of inner conscience were added through Christianity, and this composite unit of the legal, civic, moral 'person' became 'the foundation of modern political, social and legal institutions'.[12] The final transformation occurred during the eighteenth century, when the person became defined as a conscious, unique, psychological being; the modern 'self' that apparently we all live with today.[13]

Narrating the story of the self almost certainly involves locating its birth in England in the late seventeenth and eighteenth centuries. Indeed, history has emphasized that this period is traditionally understood as 'the foundation stone of the self-determining individual'.[14] Broadly speaking, attention has focused on how, in the closing decades of the seventeenth century, John Locke rendered modern selfhood conceptually possible by equating personhood with reflective thought. In his 1689 *Essay Concerning Human Understanding,* Locke defined a 'person' as a thinking entity, characterized by its inward consciousness.[15] Thanks also to the work of the philosophers Hume, Hartley and Hazlitt, the eighteenth century is also traditionally said to have given birth to a new science to support and investigate this new self – 'psychology'.[16] These and other developments are traditionally interpreted as part of a vast, all encompassing semantic reversal. As Raymond Martin and John Barresi note, Britain in the eighteenth century witnessed nothing less than 'a revolution in personal identity theory' when 'the self as immaterial soul was replaced with the self as mind':[17]

> This replacement involved movement away from substance accounts of personal identity, according to which the self is a simple persisting thing, toward relational accounts of personal identity, according to which the self consists essentially of physical and/or psychological relations among different temporal stages of an organism or person.[18]

Academics from various disciplines have embarked upon the search for the modern self in various social, political, cultural, medical, philosophical and scientific realms. Collectively, they have charted the 'rise of the individual' in many and various discourses and practices. The eighteenth-century novel has received a rather disproportionate amount of attention; it has been hailed as the cultural form 'uniquely suitable to the exploration of interiority and psychological depth', and therefore eminently suitable as an emblem for the emergence of modern selfhood.[19] Stemming from Ian Watt's influential *The Rise of the Novel* (1957), the influence of this narrative continues to be felt in the analyses of historians, literary critics and philosophers alike.[20] The history of old age has not escaped the all-pervasive influence of the individualization narrative. Susannah Ottaway's narrative charting the rise of chronological age as a key determinant in denominating someone 'old' over the course of the eighteenth century fits very neatly into this established narrative.[21] For the emphasis on a specific, individual chronological age as opposed to position in the life cycle suggests a preference for the individual, inward and particular over the collective and general. As she states herself, her findings 'can be closely connected to intellectual history', in the sense that the 'preference for autonomy corresponds with some of the most important tenets of Enlightenment philosophy'.[22] In terms of age, the 'self', one feels, inclines to measurement in chronological rather than stagistical terms.

Relating directly both to the birth of the individual and the history of age and aging is the work done by Martin Kohli on methods of measuring and conceptualizing lifetime.[23] Kohli has argued that the eighteenth century was, for the most part, characterized by 'annalistic' conception of lifetime, in which life was structured by the sequence of external historical or seasonal events. He defines this conception in opposition to the modern 'developmental' notion of lifetime that is 'organized around and by the self'.[24] The change from the former to the latter scheme – an event that Kohli locates at the end of the eighteenth century – he sees as 'parallel' to a 'fundamental change in scientific thinking', characterized by a 'transition from a spatial or categorical ordering' to a 'temporal' means of categorization. He also situates his findings within a broader historical narrative of 'individualization' and remarks that the rise of the 'self' necessarily involved 'temporalization' of life'.[25]

The most wide ranging study of personal identity in eighteenth-century England is Dror Wahrman's *The Making of the Modern Self: Identity and Culture in Eighteenth-Century England* (2004). Building on the work of Charles Taylor, Wahrman has looked beyond the exalted realms of Enlightenment philosophy and instead to the vibrant aesthetic culture of eighteenth-century England. Drawing upon various cultural forms in order to extrapolate the (often hidden) meanings of personal identity therein, Wahrman sees reflected in eighteenth-century English culture the same story of the emergence of the modern self.

By his own admission his work retells 'one of the oldest stories in the Western canon, that of the rise of modern individualism'.[26] However, Wahrman's thesis is unique in locating the emergence of the self at a very specific point in time: the closing decades of the eighteenth century. Indeed, Wahrman sees this short period as nothing short of a 'cultural revolution', characterized by the 'surprising rapidity of the transformation from one identity regime to another'.[27] His thesis of swift transition has been widely criticized by those who wish to relocate the emergence of selfhood at an earlier or later date, or by those for whom the process was slow, gradual and impossible to isolate so neatly.[28] However, these critiques of Wahrman's work seem to represent a wider problem: a focus of devoted attention upon the hallowed self and its emergence. There has been less interest in the identity regime that apparently came before it. For, it appears that the more significant implication of Wahrman's thesis is that for the first seventy or so years of the eighteenth century there was no modern self at all. Although historians and philosophers are understandably driven to explain how and when we reached our climactic sense of 'self', such narrative accounts reflect an obsession with 'modernity'. As this chapter will argue, this may lead to a myopic searching for indications of cherished 'selfhood', to the detriment of recognizing other available rubrics for comprehending identity that may be on offer. The self, we must remember, is but one mode of interpretation, and its current hegemony should not lead us to overestimate its prevalence and power in the past.

To return to Wahrman's thesis, it was not the 'self', he argues, but a different – indeed vibrantly opposite – conceptual framework that had cultural hegemony for the majority of the eighteenth century. Despite providing an account that is ostensibly all about the 'making of the modern self', it is only at the end of the century that Wahrman actually sees this self being realised. Wahrman's modern self did not emerge until late in the eighteenth century; relatively late in the day. In locating the emergence of modern selfhood in the 1770s and beyond, Wahrman has to account for another identity regime that held sway in the first seventy or so years of the eighteenth century. This he does admirably (although one cannot help suspecting that the identity regime that he describes as existing 'before the self' has been represented as something rather like the polar opposite of interior, modern selfhood). In characterizing this regime that came 'before the self', Wahrman identifies 'a consistent and wide-ranging set of assumptions that defined the meaning, significance and limits of identity up to the last two decades of the century'. This he calls the 'ancien regime of identity'.[29] As he explains, identity in the 'ancien regime' was characterized not by its interiority, but by superficiality, and by malleability. In this regime, there was a 'sense that one's 'personal identity' ... could be imagined as unfixed and potentially changeable – sometimes perceived as double, other times as sheddable, replaceable, or moldable'.[30] In the old scheme, identity was something superficial and 'socially turned', a matter of personal choice rather than biological destiny.[31] One's identity was, we might say, performed rather than experienced; and we might point to similarities between Wahrman's 'ancien regime' and the 'persona' or 'character' identified by Mauss back in 1938. Leaving aside the issue of whether the self emerged in a feat of cultural revolution, it seems that eighteenth-century England was not characterized for the most part by its self-centric modernity, but rather its pre-modernity in this respect.

The emergence of the 'self' is not the only story that can be told about identity in eighteenth-century England. Not surprisingly, historians have been keen to pick holes in this teleological modernization narrative. For example, the 'rise of the novel' orthodoxy has been seriously questioned by Deidre Lynch. Rather than seeing eighteenth-century novels as 'the prime instrument for the microscopic exploration of fevered inner consciousness', Lynch argues that characterization, not only in novels, but also in the art and theatre of eighteenth-century England was primarily generic, exhibiting types rather than individuals; personae rather than selves.[32] Work such as Lynch's suggests an important hypothesis: we ought to consider that at any one time, there may be more than one rubric for representing identity. Other notions of personhood may compete with, or just reside alongside, the 'self'. Also, the emergence of selfhood in one cultural arena does not necessitate a total eclipse of other ideas and practices. Whereas traditionally most writers have assumed that modern identity must by definition be exclusive –the changeover to modernity must be entire and all encompassing– more recently historians seem to be suggesting that modern selfhood is not incompatible with other identity forms.

Such conclusions are also present in the work of Lisa Freeman. In her *Character's Theater: Genre and Identity on the Eighteenth-Century English Stage*, Freeman describes the presence in eighteenth-century England of an alternative way of representing identity: the notion of 'character'.[33] Freeman's particular arena of study is the theatre, and she sees it as highlighting an alternative means of imagining identity that was present, although not necessarily hegemonic in eighteenth-century England. She explains that the stage in eighteenth-century culture and thought functioned to highlight the 'contradictory' and superficial aspects of personhood, and located meaning and significance 'in the contingencies and contexts that shape perception and recognition'.[34] She also draws attention to the importance of the stage in eighteenth-century culture and thought, emphasizing that its potential to influence identity concepts was anything but marginal. In Freeman's analysis, the notion of the 'character' – this 'dynamic paradigm for representing identity' – was rather like Mauss' persona, and Wahrman's 'ancien regime'. It was characterized by being capricious, malleable and socially turned. 'What the concept of character offered in the eighteenth century', Freeman writes, 'was an understanding of identity not as an emanation of stable interiority, but as the unstable product of staged contests between interpretable surfaces'.[35] In short, thanks to studies such as those of Freeman and Lynch, we have come to realize that whether or not the eighteenth century played host to the emergence of a 'modern' identity regime, alternative ways of understanding the nature of personal identity might also be present.

Overall, one result of these recent studies seems to have been to set up an imagined opposition between 'the self' and what is often represented (perhaps unnecessarily) as competing against it: whether we choose to call it the *ancien regime,* the 'persona, or the 'character'. These latter formulations have polarized and unified in the minds of scholars as something of an anti-self. The field seems to be quite bilaterally divided: on the one hand are those who see a broadly interior configuration, on the other those who see a broadly outward facing one. Although there may be some methodological prejudices and limitations here, for the purposes of this investigation, I will refer to these two historiographical constructs as the 'self' and the 'character'.

Character

It is via an elucidation of the term 'character' that this chapter hopes to add some depth to the revisionist historiography. In particular, I want to demonstrate the links between the notion of character in eighteenth-century parlance with (firstly) the body, and (secondly) the idea of aging. In order to appreciate the first of these, we need to look beneath the skin: at ideas of the character and person in the medical imagination.

In the eighteenth century, the terms 'person' and 'character' were part of medico-physiological terminology. 'Character' was one of the words used to refer to the notion of the temperament, or constitution. In Galenic terms this referred to one of the four basic types of bodily makeup resulting from a combination of bodily humours: the sanguine, cholerick, phlegmatic or melancholy. Although the Aristotelian-Galenic vision of the humoral body was on the wane in the eighteenth century, the raw concept of the temperament was certainly not.[36] As Roger Smith notes, although the language of the temperament was being gradually weaned from the language of the humors and towards the nervous configurations indicated by Cheyne, it was still very much the case that individual well-being was considered dependent on temperament.[37] Even the most progressive medical men in Western Europe ascribed to the basic idea of the temperament and most medical advice continued to be arranged around the configurations. The concept had many synonyms: in physiological and medical advice literature alone, writers employed a variety of terms freely and interchangeably, including 'temper', 'condition', 'quality', 'character', 'manner', 'disposition', 'habit' and sometimes even 'person'. In such a context, notions of 'person' and 'character' are not metaphysical abstractions, or existential puzzles, but particular formations of flesh and blood.

The physical temperament was vastly responsible for forming a person's 'character' in the sense that we mean it today. It shaped mental habits, intellectual capacity, virtues, vices, dispositions, emotional reactions, aversions and desires. One's 'character' then, in the medical imagination, was at once the physical configuration of subcutaneous substances and the consequent manifestations of these in thought, behaviour and action. This was an absolutely central tenet in early modern medicine, not merely in medical advice, but also in the emergent and ever-growing number of works on psychosomatic medicine. In his feted work of the 1760s, *On the Passions: or a Philosophical Discourse Concerning the Duty and Office of Physicians in the Management and Cure of the Disorders of the Mind*, Hieronymous David Gaubius, Professor of Chemistry at Leiden, explained how mental differences between people – character differences between people – were to be ascribed to their differing physical constitutions:

> Every particular constitution has its own distinguishing characteristic ... its own peculiar texture of the juices, its own specific course of their circulation and other corporeal operations ... so, truly, the like variety is occasioned by them in the qualifications of the mind ... For every individual body reflects a sort of self-likeness on its own mind ... for which reason the mental operations vary in different men, according to their different constitutions ... You must not therefore hope to find in every constitution an equal quickness of apprehension, exactness of judgment, sharpness of penetration, steadiness of attention, strength of memory, or liveliness of fancy. You will in vain seek for a sameness in their propensities, in their studies, in their virtues or their vices. As their bodies are diversified, so are all the abovementioned matters different in different minds.[38]

Throughout his treatise, Gaubius was at pains to emphasize how body-led characteristics really were. The crux of his work was to convince his readers that study of the mind fell within the remit of physicians rather than philosophers, and that it was the body that was largely responsible for mental disorders, foibles and attributes. In the above extract, we get the distinct sense that it is the body that not only affects the mind, but the body also that constructs the character and indeed the person. For the body is responsible for the habits, manners, studies, virtues and vices: the very constituents of character and personhood. Here, the person is a result not of mental reflection, but of their particular constellation of flesh and blood. Character was a state of body and personhood had a very material locus.

This heavily somatic notion of the person was not purely the preserve of the scientific imagination. The physical aspects of character and personhood were entrenched linguistically, as we can see by looking in Johnson's *Dictionary*. Therein, definitions of 'person' and 'character' are cross-referenced with various synonyms for the temperament. It is worth looking at some length at these definitions – although they are confusing. However, at least the following complexity should serve to underline the conceptual porosity between issues we now determine mental or physical. In the *Dictionary*, 'person' Johnson saw as synonymous with 'character'. 'Character' he defined as an 'assemblage of qualities', or 'particular constitution of the mind'. Notably, in these definitions, Johnson used the terms 'qualities' and 'constitution', both of which referenced notions of body configurations, and both of which were synonyms for the temperament. If we turn to Johnson's definition of these very terms – 'quality' and 'constitution' – we will see immediately the medico-physiological content lodged within them. 'Constitution' was to be understood as 'the corporeal frame', or 'a particular texture of parts', or 'natural qualities'. In turn, 'quality' was defined as 'disposition' or 'temper'. Again, two temperamental synonyms.

If we approach the issue from the opposite direction and start by looking at Johnson's definitions of the temperament and temper, we will also find notions of body and mind intermixed. 'Temper' Johnson defined threefold: it was foremost a 'constitution of body', secondly, 'disposition of mind' and thirdly 'constitutional frame of mind'. Here the mental and corporeal mix, and serve to confirm the influence of body on characteristics and mental activity. Along with these initial definitions came a number of further synonyms and cross-references, including 'manner', which, as Johnson explained, was a 'character of the mind'. Also implicated in the mix were 'habit' and 'condition'. The former Johnson explained could refer to 'habit of body'; the latter might mean 'natural quality of the mind', or 'temper', or 'temperament', or 'complexion'.[39] When it came to defining personhood and character therefore, Johnson's interpretations extended beyond the realms of the mental to the overtly somatic, indeed subcutaneous. Words that today carry distinctly physical overtones are integrated into concepts of personhood and character with considerable conceptual ease. Characters, persons, bodies and temperaments were semantically – and it might be suggested, conceptually – insuperable.

In Chapter 2, we encountered Gaubius noting how 'it was a trite and common observation' that people changed over the life course 'as to their understanding, reasoning, judgement, memory, inclinations, manners, and instincts'. Expanding further, he suggested that alterations in 'bodily habit' and 'complexion' could actually be definitive of personhood and that a change of temperament – more specifically through experience of different passions that characterized those temperaments – necessitated a change of 'person'.[40] Gaubius asked his readers to consider how, under the influence of 'violent passion', a man became quite unrecognizable – in fact a different person:

> Place before your eyes, gentlemen, a picture of a man fired with anger, or in great consternation through fear; captivated by love, or hurried out of himself by any other violent passion: How totally is he unlike himself in his whole body! And how impo-

tent of mind! He puts on another countenance, changes his bodily habit, varies his complexion, alters the common gestures of his limbs; his muscles are under no regulation, but act in contradiction to his will; whilst he is shaken by tremors which he cannot check; the very motions of his heart and pulse are different from what they are when natural. Digestion, nutrition, the circulation of the juices, secretions and excretions, in one word, the whole animal oeconomy is thrown into confusion. [41]

Gaubius was in no doubt that bodily change could undermine a subject's identity. 'What a change for the worse is sometimes brought on the mind of the same person even while he keeps his senses, by disorders of the body?' he asked his readers. In such a context, he suggested, 'you might almost doubt whether he be the same man or no'. Passionate and temperamental experiences had the ability to render subjects 'almost ignorant of and strangers to themselves.[42] Personhood, Gaubius suggests, could be destabilized through bodily experience. If character and personhood could be understood to reside at the level of the physical, it certainly followed that one would be different characters and different persons at different points in time, whether that be under the influence of violent passion, or in the longer term changes demanded by the life cycle.

Acting One's Age

Perhaps the best way of truly understanding the intrinsic protean and body-led nature of 'character' in eighteenth-century speech and thought is to look at a particular genre of physiological discourse that addressed the idea of character specifically: acting manuals. Flourishing at this point in time thanks to the emergence of new psycho perceptual schemes and the burgeoning significance of the passions, acting manuals may be best understood as an extension of medical literature, or indeed a psychosomatic discourse in their own right. Underwritten as they are by theories of psychosomatic self-control and passionate expression, they are emphatically not works of dramatics or aesthetics. They are works about passion and its effect on the 'character'.

It was Alan Downer, in an article of 1943, who was first to acknowledge the 'scientific' rather than aesthetic drive behind such writings; in a more recent and comprehensive study of this material, Joseph Roach endorsed the direct links between acting manuals and physiological theory.[43] Indeed, both he and Paul Goring have demonstrated the sensitivity of acting discourse to changes in physiological paradigms, noting a shift around mid-century from the more straightforward mechanistic doctrines to those with a more sensible and sensitive emphasis. Erika Fischer-Lichte has suggested that we read the historically specific presentation of the actor's body as a 'text ' composed in the 'language of emotions', thereby recognizing that actors bodies are 'culturally conditioned' in accordance with contemporary models of self-presentation.[44] Both medical advice literature and acting manuals treat of self-control and mastery over body changes, whether that is in the course of a performance, or in the course of life.

Indeed, a comparison between medical writings and acting manuals is all the more appropriate because works on acting could be written by the very same physicians who authored works of medical advice. The physician Paul Hiffernan drew upon his medical training to publish a nominally 'medical' work on the passions, yet its content and ideology was reflected in a later piece that appeared under a theatrical gloss, *The Dramatic Genius*.[45] One of the best-known examples of acting theory, *The Actor: A Treatise on the Art of Playing*, was written by John Hill, Haller's correspondent and author of two guides to health in later life.[46] This kind of overlap is hardly surprising given that acting, in eighteenth-century England, was considered a scientific phenomenon. Formulating its theory required knowledge of the passions, of physiology, of flesh and blood, and of matter in motion. '[P] Laying is a science, and is to be studied as a science', Hill explained in *The Actor*.[47] Nor would Hill necessarily have interpreted his occupations as both actor and doctor as entirely separate occupations, for in both he dealt in what Roach has felicitously termed the 'physiology of emotion'.[48] The passions were a route to bodily management, and their investigation and elucidation in this respect might cross boundaries between genres.

This literature was far from confined to a specialist market of actors. As Lisa Freeman explains, in eighteenth-century England, the significance of the theatre 'spread far beyond the theatre walls' themselves, 'through coffeehouse discussions and debates, periodical and newspaper reviews and critiques, pamphlet exchanges, and acting memoirs and biographies, both scandalous and serious'.[49] Discourse on performance theory could serve as an authoritative basis for judging actors; it could also be part of the cultivation of refined taste, an important strand of eighteenth-century polite identity.[50] The *Gentleman's Magazine* reprinted with increasing frequency insertions on the art – or science – of acting, reproduced from other specialist periodicals. *The Prompter* (1734–6) was published by Samuel Richardson, a twice-weekly twopenny half sheet combining theatrical matters with articles on social, economic and ethical issues.[51] As well the periodicals, acting discourse might also appear in other palatable forms, such as verse or biography – the poet Charles Churchill's popular, mock-heroic satire, *The Rosciad* being a typical example.[52] Additionally, histories and memoirs of the theatre – a genre that became increasingly popular from mid-century as the theatre grew in respectability – could also include insertions on acting technique.[53] In the fifty years from 1741 to 1790 nearly twenty of these 'histories' were published.[54]

Although such discourse focused on body changes in a specific spatial and temporal arena – the stage – the significance of the physiological and passionate processes discussed therein were by no means limited to drama. Nor is the body discussed in acting theory considered to be a professional performing body that is somehow different and more artificial than a normal body. The 'actor' therein always stands for the 'actor' in a far broader sense – the social actor. Within acting manuals and the attendant discourse, it is typically implied that social intercourse itself is a form of acting and that daily life is a kind of performance of the passionate body. As Boswell noted in his own foray into acting theory, a series of essays in *The London Magazine* in 1770, 'It is surely not only an object of taste to study theatrical representations, but it may be a matter of very curious philosophical enquiry', for the experience of getting into character was something 'experienced by many men in the common intercourse of life'.[55] Both acting theory and medical advice advocate social improvement via the successful 'manipulation of the body'.[56] Although unrelated in form, these two genres are related by their interest in matters of human agency and body change and in how embodied identity may be subject to laws of mind over matter.

When it came to discussing ideas about 'character', character changes or getting into character, acting manuals relied heavily on notions of the temperament and constitution. In his 1741 *History of the English Stage*, Edmund Curll explained that acting was essentially a question of comprehending and representing different 'characters' amongst humankind. The difference between characters, Curll stated – both on the stage and in real life – was essentially corporeal matter. Curll wrote in medical idiom, also employing rather a lot of the temperamental synonyms found in Johnson's *Dictionary*. The following extract – admittedly somewhat confusing to our modern eyes – is testament to the inherently somatic dimension of character in the eighteenth-century imagination as well as to the vast catalogue of terms that might be employed to give this emphasis. The actor's art, Curll explained, might be comprehended thus:

> Now what he [the actor] represents is Man in his various Characters, Manner and Passions ... He must perfectly express the Quality and Manners of the Man whose Person he assumes. That is, he must know how his Manners are compounded, and from thence know the several Features, as I may call them, of his Passions. An *Actor* must ... carry the Person in all his Manners and Qualities with him in every Action and Passion; he must transform himself into every Person he represents ... Sometimes he is to be a Lover, and know not only all the soft and tender Addresses of one, but what are proper to the Character of Him who is in Love, whether he be ... a hot or fiery Man, or of more moderate and flegmatic Constitution, and even the Degrees of the Passion he is possessed with. Sometimes he is to represent a choleric, hot and jealous Man ... then he must be thoroughly acquainted with all the Motions and Sentiments productive of those Motions of the Feet, Hands and Looks of such a Person all dejected and bending under the Extremities of Grief and Sorrow; which changes the whole Form and Appearance of him in the Representation, as it does really in Nature.[57]

The sheer number of terms Curll uses here is confounding. It is unclear which terms refer to abstract entities and which to material or physiological configurations – or indeed whether Curll envisages a distinction between physical and metaphysical at all. A 'person', for example is seen to be something that may be achieved through conscious transformation, as long the actor is familiar with the 'manners and qualities' required to make that person. Curll also makes specific reference to the four humours: embodied in the hot and fiery lover, and the man of moderate and 'flegmatic Constitution' is the old language of Galen and Aristotle. It seems that Curll expected his readers to understand the notion of 'character' and 'person' as material configurations of flesh and blood, and that it was entirely fitting to discuss his ideas about characters in somatic terms. It is no wonder he suggested that the actor 'ought to have an Insight into Moral Philosophy', for it would be necessary to appreciate the 'different Compositions of the Manners' and the passions 'springing from them'. As Curll seems to have suggested, comprehending characters and persons required looking into their physiological, chemical 'composition'.[58] His belief that characters were essentially a product of humoral blends is suggested finally by his comment that 'various Appearances in the Looks and Actions' might be put down to 'various Mixtures'.[59] Mixtures, that is, of elemental essences beneath the skin.

Writers of acting manuals often discussed how it was that actors might learn to appreciate and represent differences between characters. In order to furnish their discussions, writers resorted to the language of the temperament. The celebrated Garrick leant heavily on temperamental imagery in his own exposition of 'character'. 'The only Way to arrive at *great Excellency* in *Characters* of *Humour*,' he wrote,

> Is to be very conversant with *Human Nature*, ... by this Way you will more accurately discover the *Workings of Spirit* (or what other Physical Terms you please to call it) upon the different *Modifications* of *Matter* ... let him [the actor] be introduc'd into the World, be conversant with *Humours* of every Kind'[60]

At first glance it appears that Garrick's reference to 'Characters of Humour' is a reference to roles in comical plays. But, given the content of the extract, it becomes apparent that the term has a very useful double meaning. For 'characters of humour' may refer also to the characteristics arising from differing temperaments: different configurations of the humours in a human body. This is confirmed by Garrick's second use of the term '*Humours*' in the final line, where it is surely meant to convey the panoply of temperamental differences between people: society is a cultural patchwork of '*Humours* of every Kind'. The different 'modifications of matter' is a reference to the physiological differences, the different constitutions or temperaments in different human bodies. Garrick himself was clearly no stranger to developments in physiology; he had cultivated a working knowledge of material mechanism and rendered it serviceable to his own theory of acting. It seems that he was equally attuned to the body dimensions involved in characterization. The double meanings in his language, the inherent theatricality in notions of temperamental bodies and the inherent temperamental meanings inherent in notions of characters – give a now forgotten materiality and tangibility to these discussions. Characterization in the theatre, as in the course of life, was a somatic experience.

The temperamental body is also present in the language contemporaries used to applaud and authenticate judgments about successful characterization. The anonymous correspondent who praised Garrick so highly in the *Gentleman's Magazine* in 1743 interpreted the actor's amazing protean ability as the achievement of real changes of 'temper' and 'habit'. Having already championed Garrick's apparent fittingness for demanding roles in the tragic genre, the devotee then effused about his striking ability to mould himself to roles of quite the opposite nature: 'In *low Comedy* the same Man keeps the Spectators in continual *good Humour*', he enthused, 'and his *Face* is as well suited to the *Temper* he is to express as if his *Soul* ever wore *another Habit*.'[61] References to the 'temper' and 'habit' suggest a real power of material metamorphosis, for in changing characters, Garrick changes 'temper' and 'habit'. Being able to change these is what effects characterization. Moreover, somatic change is not achieved in Garrick alone, but also occurs in the bodies of those who watch him, for, according to this correspondent, Garrick 'keeps the Spectators in continual *good Humour*'. When celebrating a successful characterization in eighteenth-century terms, it seems necessary to resort to notions of the temperamental body. In acting manuals, the temperamental character is referenced ubiquitously to demonstrate the reality, the materiality and the power of the theatrical experience.

This brings us to a particular issue that has fascinated historians of both identity and the eighteenth-century theatre. Namely, why was it that eighteenth-century commentators so often insisted that actors *really* became the character they represented for the course of the performance? Why did getting into character, in an eighteenth-century context, apparently involve a real change of identity? Belief in this literal transformation was expressed freely and ubiquitously in acting manuals, and the issue was given extended philosophical analysis by James Boswell in a series of essays in the *London Magazine*. What seems plausible in this context is the presence of a notion of character that was material, temperamental and inherently protean. One which brought with it implicit associations with life course changes in temperament, passionate experiences, manners and habits. That contemporaries might have been referencing such a notion of 'character' is suggested by Samuel Derrick's discussion in his *General View of the Stage*. When Derrick was celebrating this exact power; the ability of the consummate actor to 'make a temporary renunciation of himself' and 'forget, if possible, his own identity' the explanation Derrick reached for was that of the temperamental character:[62]

> To do justice to his character, he must not only strongly impress it on his own mind, but make a temporary renunciation of himself and all his connections in common life, and for a few hours consign all his private joys and griefs to oblivion; forget, if

possible, his own identity. How difficult, and yet how requisite the task! He must put on the character with the habit, and assume the air, look, language, and action of the person he represents, till his imagination, quite absorpt in the extensive idea, influences his whole frame; is visible in every glance of the eye, every air of his countenance. Thus all his powers will sometimes swell with the most violent transports of rage, and again dissolve away by an insensible gradation into the most placed calm and serenity. This is not so much acting as being an original; and the Actor who has attained this has reached the summit of his art.[63]

A successful transformation, Derrick explained, required the actor to 'put on the character with the habit, and assume the air, look, language, and action of the person he represents'. Firstly, we might observe that Derrick employed the terms 'character' and 'habit', terms that, in Johnson's estimation, could be understood as synonymous. Ostensibly the use of 'habit' here refers to the actor's costume – the clothes themselves – but the dual meaning and juxtaposing of terms is both confounding and suggestive. Putting on *both* the character *and* the habit at least suggests that costuming itself is inadequate, and that a more physical transformation is required. And, to emphasize the somatic dimension of such a change, Derrick confirms that it is via the physical manifestations – the air, look, language and action – that this 'character' change will be known. In acknowledging 'how difficult' this change was, Derrick suggested that it was something physical – something above and beyond mental identification alone. If we suppose that Derrick, and indeed other commentators, were referencing notions of the temperamental character, and that in so doing they were implicitly referencing body changes that attended progress through life, these claims make more sense. Changes in temperament, like changes on the stage were psychosomatic experiences; in both cases, character was located in the body and changed as a result of that body's metamorphosis.

There was little conceptual distinction between 'character' changes on the stage and character changes through life. Because the eighteenth-century concept of character was so material and so life-course orientated, and because acting involved real physical changes of the same temperamental nature, acting and aging were conceptually closer than we might imagine. At least, the two concepts were separated by differences of degree rather than kind. Acting and aging – body changes that we now see as entirely separate types of occurrences – one feigned, transitory and outward facing, the other biological, inward, permanent and inherent – are actually linked in the eighteenth-century imagination by the notion of the temperamental character. We can't help supposing that when contemporaries read about actors making shifts from one habit, one character to another, it must have carried overtones of real life course transitions between 'characters' or 'persons' in real life.

It is hardly surprising that the terminology used to discuss life and one's progress through it in eighteenth-century England was overtly and explicitly theatrical. The idea that progress through life was in steps – discrete and significant rites of passage as opposed to steady linear development – placed emphasis on tangible breaks and changes in roles. As we saw in Chapter 2, it made physiological sense to anticipate that one might play a series of different characters as the life cycle progressed. Life was, after all, measured in 'stages'. The theatre was a singularly significant trope in eighteenth-century thought, and theatrical metaphors provided ways of making sense of daily societal interaction. As Philip Thicknesse wrote in his *Valetudinarians Bath Guide* of 1780,

> by the time a man arrives at three score, he has had such frequent opportunities of examining the wires and mechanism of the great shew (THE WOLRD) and thereby discovering, how the tricks are performed, that the entertainment ceases.[64]

As Ronald Paulson demonstrated in 1976, theatricality was a metaphor of growing importance throughout the eighteenth century, one that was endorsed explicitly for its peculiar suitability by Addison in the *Spectator*.[65] Theatrical allusions were not merely blithe euphemisms for the transience or arbitrariness of social life. In the words of Lisa Freeman, in eighteenth-century England, 'theatricality [was] the governing metaphor of social life and the primary filter of psychic perception'.[66] Indeed, as David Marshall states, 'the figure of theatre provides a significant cultural paradigm for eighteenth-century English culture'.[67]

Marshall has drawn attention to the 'inherently theatrical' nature of eighteenth-century doctrines of social interaction, particularly Adam Smith's ideology of sympathy.[68] For Smith, Marshall argues, along with other writers such as Hutcheson and Hume, 'moral philosophy has entered the theatre' and sympathy 'is designed to address the theatrical character of the way people face each other in the world'.[69] John Brewer argues that theatricality was definitive of social relations feeling the pressures of a new economic climate. 'Manners' were adopted as a form of social regulation for volatile relations, a way of controlling and minimizing risk by codified behaviour.[70] In the 'increasingly performative' nature of eighteenth-century England, theatre was the favoured metaphor for interpreting one's journey through life as well as one's experience of aging.[71] Perhaps it is not surprising to find that Aaron Hill, who wrote the extended prose poem on *The Art of Acting*, also penned one entitled *The Distinction of Ages,* a piece meditating on the seven stages of life and the great differences of character attendant upon them. The poem characterized each life stage via its passionate and temperamental experiences, using the Galenic idiom. From twenty-eight until thirty-five, Hill explained, 'Life's *gay fire* / Sparkles, Sparkles, burns loud, and flames, in *fierce desire*'. Whereas, 'At *fifty six* cool *reason* reigns, intire / Then, life burns *steddy*, and with *temp'rate fire*'.[72] The poem not only cements the body centric element of these changes, but their swift juxtaposition recalls a suggestion of the swiftness with which an actor might shed one role and begin the next. Actors became different characters over the course of their performance in the same conceptual and physiological ways that ordinary people became different characters over the life course: via changes in the temperament. When Boswell commented that 'MR GARRICK exhibits in his own person such a variety of characters', it was in a sense no different to the variety of characters one might experience over the life course.[73] The only difference (and why Garrick was considered so talented) was that he was able to bring them forth on demand and experience them simultaneously: by training his body and exercising an extraordinary (and possibly detrimental) level of self-control. Actors, if we remember from Chapter 3, were not considered long livers on account of the extraordinary wear and tear to which they subjected their bodies.

Contemporaries were all too ready to point to the fact that experience of passion on stage was of exactly the same nature as the experience of passion in real life. The stage was 'the seat of passion', as Curll put it, but the 'representation', of passion here was essentially equal to what happened 'really in Nature'.[74] Henry Fielding, diverting briefly to make 'a Comparison between the World and the Stage', in *Tom Jones,* knew that passionate experience in real life and on the stage was of exactly the same nature, and by extension, regulating the passions in daily life might just as well to be understood as acting. The passions, Fielding wrote, were the 'Managers and Directors' of the Theatre of Life, and 'often force Men upon Parts, without consulting their Judgment, and sometimes without any Regard to their Talents'.[75] The temporary body changes spoken of in context of acting discourse have to be understood in context of body changes more broadly. Not only those temporary body changes brought about by the passions, but those changes over the longue durée – the changes that constitute the aging of the body over lifetime. Acting and aging were both temperamental issues and as such they both helped shape the meaning of the character and the person.

Conclusion

This chapter has used the concept of aging to investigate formations of identity in eighteenth-century England. Although historians have identified the protean nature of 'character' in an eighteenth-century cultural context, they have failed to appreciate how this could be attributed to its fundamental links with the body, particularly the temperament and aging body. Investigating personhood and character via the body, and especially the aging body, allows us to see these important and frequently overlooked features of identity concepts in eighteenth-century England. Unlike our notion of character today, the eighteenth-century concept was inherently unstable. The value of character is not to be found solely in various cultural forms or practices like the theatre or the novel, not just a rubric which, is to be found 'in the drama and on the stage', but which was played out via the body by every person in the theatre of life.[76] The protean nature of character was embedded at a physical, somatic (and perhaps a 'natural') level.

It must be emphasized that these particular understandings of personhood and character were not necessarily exclusive. At any one time there may be various rubrics available for comprehending notions of the person or character. Writers who conceived of the character in somatic, temporal terms did not necessary have no notion of an inner consciousness. The presence of the temperamental character does not automatically negate the presence of a more modern, interior sense of self. Rather the vision of the temperamental character was, it seems, an accepted and important way of comprehending identity. However, some aspects of this conception of character do seem incompatible with notions of the modern self. When Locke rendered modern selfhood possible by equating it with conscious thought, he drew attention to stability over time. What made a person a person was the fact he or she *was* the same person when his or her body changed. Locke's notion of personhood required temporal extension and, as Martin and Barresi confirm, that is still the precondition for 'selfhood' today. Selfhood resides in 'physical and/or psychological relations among different temporal stages of an organism or person'.[77] The temperamental character by contrast, was inherently protean and unstable. It altered in accordance with the changes thrust upon it by societal rites of passage, violent passions and theatrical flights of fancy. Quite simply, the prevalence and persistence of the two concepts of temperament and the life cycle, seen in synch as they habitually were, were concepts largely incompatible with the modern sense of self. Both presumed a capacity for step change, movement between roles and characters, the idea that different characters or persons could be present in the same body over the life course. Surely the notion of a modern 'self' is in fact opposed to the notion of a life cycle and more inclined to require the concept of a lifelong aging process, probably measured in chronological years. As both Susannah Ottaway and Martin Kohli have pointed out, measuring age in chronological years and the 'temporalization' of life – practices which they have independently identified as gaining muster towards the end of the eighteenth-century – are practices that appear to depend on a more modern, interior, individual identity formations. Whether or not these particular practices are incompatible with notions of the temperamental character is debatable and remains to be seen. Yet certainly the notion of the temperamental character was not built on the same fundamental premises as Locke's seminal configuration.

Using the concept of aging to investigate identity has drawn attention to two historiographical issues in particular. In these extracts, we have seen the presence of the body in identity concepts where it has been lost or forgotten today. By drawing attention to the temperamental aspect of 'character' in the eighteenth-century imagination, it was possible to demonstrate how eighteenth-century identity concepts were still heavily psychosomatic as well as purely mental or abstract. We have become attuned to thinking about the person as something above mere flesh and blood; we think about character as being a set of mental dispositions. 'Character' is, according to the *Oxford English Dictionary,* the 'mental and moral qualities distinctive to an individual'. We recognize, for sure, that the body can be a place where aspects of identity are displayed, but we tend not to appreciate that the physical body something that perhaps *is* character, rather than just being a prop in making it. The sacred sense of 'self' – so closely attuned as it is to concepts of rationality – seems to be located above and beyond corporeality. But, in an eighteenth-century context, 'character' and 'person', as well as a whole host of other synonyms, cannot be understood without the body. It seems fitting to use an expression of Karl Figlio's here: the 'body', in these imaginings, 'is an inseparable extension of the self.'[78]

In an eighteenth-century context, notions of character and personhood were, I suggest, inherently protean. Their links with the temperament and the life cycle were absolutely central to their meaning and definition. Physiologically, everyone experienced being different characters, perhaps different 'persons' throughout life as a matter of course. Rather than being a stable identity concept, 'character' implicitly referenced notions of diachronic change. Indeed, we might suggest that the real value of the concept of character came from the fact that it could reference the possibility of long-term change in human experience. To talk about the 'character' in an eighteenth-century context was to draw attention to the changeability of identity. We tend to want to locate interiority with permanence; today the self and the person seems the bit that hopefully, reassuringly stays the same despite the caprice and decline of the flesh. But eighteenth-century notions of personhood were more intrinsically about change, predicated on notions of bodily caprice.

Without the perspective brought about by studying aging, scholars cannot acknowledge a very simple reflection of the 'character' in one of the most basic tropes of early modern thought. Characters changed over the course of the life cycle. One's experience of 'aging' in the eighteenth century was one grand example of how mutable personhood could be. When thinking about aspects of identity, historians tend to think in static rather than developmental terms; it is rarely acknowledged that identities have a diachronic aspect. This chapter has stressed the importance of change over time in the construction of identities. Identities are not about permanence, but constantly under construction. Much historical research into identity has regarded embodied identity as being rather static over lifetime. Yet it seems that the defining aspect of pre-modern identity – its mutability and malleability – requires the dimensions of time, age and body change in order to be fully appreciated. In conducting his grand tour of identity in eighteenth-century English culture, Wahrman considered gender, race, class, even the distinction between animals and humans, but not age. However it appears that it is an important way of understanding how eighteenth-century people might have defined themselves. Age and aging were written into eighteenth-century identity concepts at an etymological, physiological, medical and cultural level. Perhaps historians should pay more attention to them when investigating past constructions of identity.

CONCLUSION

This final chapter draws together the conclusions from the six chapters and suggests how the findings herein might help shape research in the future. Given that the method here has incorporated approaches from social history, medical history, the history of ideas and the history of the body, I offer some comments about the value of bringing together these lines of enquiry and situate the work within the historiography of each. Finally, considering some contemporary ideas about age, aging and identity, I ask whether current research into aging can benefit from looking at the pre-modern ideas outlined in this study.

When it comes to exploring how aging was understood in the eighteenth century, this work has attempted to characterize a multitude of ideas, illustrating their complexity and flexibility. This was a period of epistemological inclusivity, when it was possible to interpret age and the aging body in a number of modal registers, and when ideas about aging stretched way beyond the remit of medicine or physiology. The process that we now recognize as aging was something of a composite of ideas in the eighteenth century. Aging involved the interweaving of notions of health and the body, disease and decay, good and bad, spirituality, cosmology, character, self-control, sociability, and forces of nature. An eighteenth-century aging process (to speak anachronistically) was a patchwork of experiences on many levels; a thing capricious; a relationship with the world that was not led first and foremost by chronological or biological time.

In general, the conclusions reached here do support Ottaway's judgment that, for the most part, old age was measured culturally rather than chronologically. However, this study has not represented a chronological narrative in line with Ottaway's findings. Ottaway has charted how increasing importance was placed on actual chronological age as its determinant over the course of the century.[1] We must concede that chronology – in fact just the basic awareness of time – was gathering importance as the century progressed, and this manifested in several behaviours and practices. As Robert Poole has demonstrated, the concept of historical time was being 'grasped with increasing alacrity by the middling sorts in society', the techniques of measuring it were becoming ever more sophisticated, the practice of measuring it was growing ever more widespread, and the means of measuring it, in the form of clocks and pocket-watches, ever more widely owned.[2]

Similarly, developments such as the accurate measurement of longitude and the growth of regular fast stage-coach services made it easier to divide up time and travel in predictable segments. The potential to master time was evident in the reformation of the calendar in 1752, which brought Britain in line with the Continent. These developments, when contextualized within Ottaway's narrative, provide the background as to why chronological age may have begun to figure more pertinently in the minds of officials and regulators – even at parish level – as the century progressed. However, such trends have not been reflected in the areas considered in this book. It is important to note that Ottaway's work is not a study of aging, but a study of old age and its definition. It seems entirely plausible to imagine that chronological determinants may have been on the increase without this necessarily impacting upon ideas about aging itself, what caused it, or how to manage it. Measuring old age is a very different endeavour to explaining why the body ages, or suggesting how the aging body can be manipulated for social effect. As such then, this study does not appear incompatible with Ottaway's findings; rather it offers a different perspective on 'aging'.

The history of age and aging intersects with many different historical disciplines. This study has focused on concepts, language, medicine, bodies and identities, but there are other ideological frameworks that could be used to research the subject. Histories of aging could be presented through various heuristic lenses: political ideas, legal developments, demography, spirituality, or the history of time. Yet it is hoped that the focus of the preceding chapters is salient in that it represents concerns of the unique historical moment. In the new consumer society, aging was a phenomenon over which a considerable amount of commercial literature was produced, and it was a newly profitable commodity to be exploited. Aging was visible in the eighteenth-century; more anti-aging solutions emerged than ever before, some of them ingenious, some bizarre. At this point in time, aging was mostly understood as a problem to be solved; it was not the social / demographic problem we face today, but an intriguing conundrum that could be engaged with in various social, medical, philosophical, chemical and spiritual ways.

We have encountered aging in the Enlightenment realm of the social: pliant to the demands of polite sociable interaction, and itself a means of disseminating acceptable behaviour and conduct. Aging was made into a sociable issue, and aging body management could become a shared practice in which all self-conscious health consumers could engage. Like politeness, aging was something that needed to be engaged with at an individual level, yet its benefits were to be realised and enjoyed in a social arena. Aging could afford a certain amount of experiment and even enjoyment: life might be extended by inhaling the breath of healthy young virgins, or at very least enjoying pleasant, cheerful company. Still, the aging body could also be a site for the representation of all that was nasty and ugly in the world, and alongside expressions of faith in progress came expressions of anxiety about the limits of man's control over his ultimate mortality.

Deserving particular mention in this short conclusion is cheerfulness. Within the parameters of this study, it has already been possible to see the particular frequency in which the term arises, and the particular significance it was afforded in contemporary writings. Although it was a concept with especial value for aging, the qualities that it referenced and the philosophy that it represented had a far broader significance. Cheerfulness had a unique ability to represent particular cultural values – in much the same ways that the term 'polite' became a slogan for the dissemination of middle-class behavioural codes. It has also been suggested that cheerfulness might be understood in context of contemporary theories of social interaction: a tangible force in its own right like the 'sympathy' envisaged by the century's ontologists. The distinctive values inherent in the eighteenth-century concept of cheerfulness suggest an area ripe for further historical research. We may even go as far as claiming that cheerfulness represents an important alternative paradigm: a challenge to the hegemony of politeness.

As far as scientific paradigms are concerned, eighteenth-century writings on aging are characterized by the inclusivity and flexibility of explanatory schemes on offer. The aging body could be imagined as a bucket of humours, a hydraulic machine, a bundle of sensitive nerves, or a pick-and-mix selection of all of them. Although separable in theory, paradigms were not watertight or exclusive, and ideas overlapped in medical advice. This co-existence of paradigms old and new is distinctive and may be considered to compound the notion of the eighteenth century as sandwiched between the pre-modern and modern worlds. However, whereas this inclusivity may belie a gradual shift in explanatory frameworks, it emphatically does not appear that *ideas* were changing very much. Whereas the eighteenth century is often presented as characterized by gradual secularization and 'biologization', the sources examined in this study do not suggest that the aging body was subject to modernizing thought. From a history of the body perspective, the 'body' presented in this study is a flexible, malleable and porous body. It is a body that responds in kind to affective phenomena in the outside world, a body that alters physically via passionate and emotional experience. Although these are all characteristics that might be attributed to the continuing legacy of the 'old' body, it seems that they travelled across physiological paradigms. When it came to identifying the causes of aging, new paradigms actually reinforced old beliefs. In medical advice, a combination of old and new ideas were collated to create a picture of an aging body which was highly responsive to external phenomena; which 'wore out' on account of its historical, geographical and social surroundings and subjective experience. Even in the most 'scientific' of imaginations, aging continued to be described as the result of external forces upon the body. Although Boerhaave and Haller described the physical manifestations of aging in more scientific ways, they still located the affective phenomena at a socio-cultural level, insisting that aging was a highly contingent experience. Ultimately then, although we can read these texts paradigmatically, it is not the paradigms that are important. Focusing on the amalgamation and development of explanatory frameworks is less important than acknowledging the continuity of ideas contained within them.

In eighteenth-century England, aging was largely understood to be a matter of personal choice. Eighteenth-century writers understood the aging body as a product of lived experience and sought to enable their readership to create and manage that product. Across paradigms, ownership of the physical self involved wearing it out at one's own idiosyncratic rate. As a consequence, the degree of agency imagined for the human agent over the aging body was extremely generous, if not hopeful. What we see in these texts are not merely sentiments of encouragement to engage with the aging body and alleviate suffering, but the laying open of an aging body which is in itself understood to be highly interactive and ripe to be mastered. The self-conscious self-fashioner is offered a tangible reach beneath the skin. In the terms currently used in the historiography of embodied identity, we might say that aging, in the eighteenth-century imagination, was largely conceived to be a matter of choice rather than destiny.

Of course, the championing of human agency over the body must be understood in the climate of rational, democratic healthcare from which these publications emerged. The sentiment may be partially accounted for by the call to arms of these democratizing physicians who wished to 'lay open' medical therapeutics and empower their readers for the benefit of a progressive, healthy, Enlightened society. Buchan wanted to empower his readers by showing them how they could create their own medicines with readily available foodstuffs and seasonings. Yet this rationalizing, democratizing impetus that characterized eighteenth-century medical advice generally does not seem to be an adequate explanation for the championing of agency over the *aging* body. The inclusion of the aging body in medical advice literature – that is, the *recognition* of the aging body as a site for management – was not merely the logical extension of a historically and culturally specific vogue. If we are to understand why physicians preached management of the aging body, we need to look deeper than the particularities of the discourse in which they were expressed: not just to the cultural and commercial drivers that funded such sentiments, but also to the fundamental epistemes that enabled them. Rather than just interpreting these physicians' views of the aging body as shaped by – and for – commercial, prescriptive literature, it is important to note that at this point in time it was conceptually viable to see aging as malleable. In fact, the great potential envisaged for the human agent at this point in time can surely account for the great number of medical advice works which appeared in the course of the century, as well as the vast numbers that included promises of 'long life' in their titles. Long life was possible, plausible and newly visible: publications reflected rather than merely created this belief. Thanks to a unique combination of factors – a flexible epistemological framework, the presence of both new and old ways of interpreting the body, and a burgeoning print culture straining to meet the demands of a health-hungry society – agency over the aging body was championed in proportions that would have been, and would be, impossible before or since.

It would be historiographically unforgivable to talk about agency over the body without making reference to the position and power of the medical establishment. These physicians may have had a rationalizing, democratic impetus, but there was a prescriptive, defining and confining influence being exerted too. Certain behaviours and practices were positively scorned in medical advice, for example academic or 'studious' pursuits. These ideas could be 'naturalised' when articulated through the language of sensibility and nervous strain. Equally, the suggested behaviours and practices in medical advice were shaped by – and shaped – dominant codes of conduct. These books helped stigmatize the undesirable and set the standards for what was correct, virtuous and socially acceptable. However, we might argue that the methods suggested were a means of augmenting individual agency. As well as traditional regimen, therapies for the aging body included sociable interaction, diverting amusements and even inhaling the breath of healthy young women. Hence, eighteenth-century medical writers do not present the aging body as a problem to be solved via exclusively medical means, and certainly not via direct contact with medical practitioners. The 'cure' for the aging body – as the rhetoric of cheerfulness suggests – was just as likely to be located in the realm of the social as in that of the medical establishment.

From a methodological point of view, this book draws attention to the pitiful neglect with which 'aging' has been treated as a tool of analysis for investigating identity. Race, class and gender – other aspects of embodied identity – are now standard heuristic tools, but age and aging have been studiously ignored, much to the detriment of our understanding of 'identity' in the past. Chapter Five exemplified this neglect, showing how in the historiography of masculinity to date, the age criterion has been almost entirely absent. Although many studies on aspects of eighteenth-century masculinity have appeared in the last ten years, none of them have had much to say about how age affects masculinity, or whether hegemonic constructions of masculinity allowed for the inclusion of aging men. The chapter concluded by noting how distinct older men seemed to be from their younger counterparts. Old age required a specific set of behaviours that were clearly quite opposed to those considered appropriate for men in earlier life. This reinforces the argument for the continued hegemony of the life cycle as a sense-making strategy. As we saw in Chapter Two, eighteenth-century writings on aging continued to assume that because everyone went through different stages in life, everyone experienced being different 'characters' at each of those different stages. Of course it followed that certain identities would come naturally to each stage, and that certain behaviours would befit those certain identities. Although scholars have argued for the etymological development of the term 'masculinity' in the eighteenth century (the shift away from 'masculinity' being associated with a certain life stage), those who wrote about aging in the eighteenth century actually maintained that old age was a discrete stage of life.

The idea of aging as identity is ripe for deconstruction. Not least because like those other kinds of identity played out on the body, aging is an aspect of identity that has a mixture of biological and cultural aspects, aspects of choice and aspects of destiny. Historians are used to deconstructing historical notions of gender and race, and in so doing, the normal heuristic method is to look at the relative balance of 'natural' versus 'cultural' factors inherent in these concepts. This broadly Foucauldian analysis, honed by Laqueur and more recently employed by Wahrman, basically involves drawing out the interplay of biological and cultural factors forming the definitions of gender, race or class, and understanding the degree to which individual identity may be said therefore to be a matter of choice or destiny. Undoubtedly, age and aging are more nebulous aspects of identity than race or gender, and it may be presumptuous to assume that concepts of aging can be divided neatly into biological or cultural formations. Whereas the two concepts of gender and sex allow distinction between the biological and the cultural, age and aging do not have a comparable pairing of concepts to work with. There is the modern gerontological distinction between chronological and cultural age, but, as we discovered in Chapter One, this may be a limited heuristic framework for historical analysis. Moreover, this is a means of categorizing 'age' itself, rather than the more amorphous notion of 'aging'.

Still, it is worth thinking about whether 'aging identity' or 'age identity' can be deconstructed along broadly nature/ culture lines in historical enquiry. We might now briefly scrutinize the findings in this book in such a fashion. We can consider the ideas we have encountered in preceding chapters and use these conclusions to think about 'aging' as an aspect of identity made up of a balance of natural and cultural components. Chronological age, in the eighteenth-century was not an important category of identity. It was not an adequate, definitive standard of explanation, but more of an empty category, which only reflected or supported the truths inherent in cultural understandings of age. The word itself – 'age' – carried fewer associations with human experience than it does today, and as such talking about 'age' in the eighteenth-century was not necessarily to speak of how old someone was, or about one's experience of aging. 'Age' was more likely to be a measurement of historical time rather than individual development. Furthermore, when applied as a subjective judgement it was more likely to refer to the state of visible decay on a human body; one's 'age' in this context was largely dependent on one's state of health. The identity that 'age' conferred in this sense was a physical, changeable one, rather than a biological one. And it was also highly subjective: it relied on the personal and intuitive judgement of whoever was looking, and not upon quantifiable, unalterable facts.

Age identity could reflect the individual's moral, social and behavioural choices. Nowhere could this be better demonstrated than through the rhetoric of cheerfulness. As polite and cheerful behaviours were championed as having anti-aging properties, an aging body could reflect an individual's capacity for successful sociable interaction and benign restraint. Those who were most cheerful aged well. By extension, the implication was that that those who were aging well were cheerful, polite, socially desirable and correct. In Godwin's Utopian vision, age identity would reflect rational capacity, for longevity was a marker of the achievement of psychosomatic self-mastery. The sense of identity conferred by age was further complicated by the fact that the aging body was seen as an incarnation of other metaphysical judgements: the aging body could function as a site for reading moral or spiritual probity. In the Biblical scheme, aging was not an original or therefore 'natural' phenomenon, it was punishment for Sin – something that Wesley was all too keen to remind his readers at the outset of his popular medical text. Spiritual advice infiltrated medical advice, and accounts of patriarchal longevity sat cheek by jowl with medical aphorisms. In a broader sense, the juxtaposition between youth and age could be called upon to represent the more basic division between good and bad. Age identity then, was complex: not only was it a barometer of psychosomatic health, it also had the ability to indicate moral standing, intellectual ability and spiritual probity.

That the identity conveyed by an aging body was more a matter of personal choice rather than destiny is further suggested by the fact that aging was sometimes described as surmountable. Along with references to the possibility of 'growing young again' came various tales of rejuvenation in popular literature and medical advice. Cohausen's chemical satire of 1743 suggested that the transfer of breath might involve 'borrowing fresh Spirits' from the young breath donor. This he described as 'enjoy[ing] two Sorts of Life'.[3] Indeed, looking more closely at the language Cohausen uses to describe what is happening as the breath takes effect we see that this process of rejuvenation involves an actual transfer of the 'Quality' of youth, so that the aged subject – the eponymous 'Hermippus' – takes on another, or a second identity:

> When the blooming *Thysbe*, whom the Graces adorn, and the Muses instruct, converges with the good old Hermippus, her Youth invigorates his Age ... borrowing

> fresh Spirits from the lovely Thysbe, what Wonder that he, who enjoys two Sorts of Life, should live twice as long as another Man?'[4]

Cohausen seems to have introduced the possibility of one's age being an aspect of identity that can be borrowed or shared. Rejuvenescence, in this context, is presented as the (temporary) assumption of another identity. The *Gentleman's Magazine* also picked up on this trope, stating that if such a breath transfer was possible, 'we may even go so far as to say, that with his own he enjoys a borrow'd Life; and therefore we need not wonder that he should *last* twice as long as other Men'.[5] This kind of 'borrowing' or sharing of experiences and qualities was not just metaphorical but a physical possibility in the minds of the century's ontologists. Whether it be through pleasant company, human nature, sympathy, electricity, or breath, aspects of identity or personality were not necessarily bounded within the individual, but shareable and transferable. There is, perhaps, a suggestion in these texts that the experience of (or perhaps we may say the essence of) aging could do likewise.

If modern social theorists are to be believed, in the twenty-first century we do have biologically skewed age gazes. We are, apparently, blissfully ignorant about quite how 'aged by culture' we are. The current movement towards 'biosociality' in sociology and gerontology attempts to redefine the categories of 'natural' and 'cultural' aging. As the sociologist Stephen Katz explains, 'biosocial' discourses question the ontological role played by 'nature' in the aging process, asking 'was the natural ever all that natural?' and suggesting that cultural age is itself an entirely 'natural' category.[6] To different ends, the feminist critic, Margaret Morganroth Gullette, has theorized that age-systems are so socially constructed and so embedded that it is impossible to determine what is natural.[7] In her book, *Aged by Culture,* Gullette points out that 'aging' in twenty-first century parlance typically refers to 'age on the body'. 'Traditionally', she writes, aging has been 'considered a continuum in which visible change is driven by involuntary mechanisms'; a position that consigns us to being 'passive victims of 'aging processes'. Now, she claims, we need to emphasize the 'active' aspects of aging such as 'intentional changes of behaviour ... and will'.[8]

Notwithstanding Gullette's overtly politicized urge, her hopes for the future experience of aging are actually quite pertinent to some of the findings in this study. Not least her methodological points about using age as a heuristic tool for investigating identity. Gullette draws attention to the fact that intellectual theorizing in the early twenty-first century tended to ignore the diachronic aspects of personal identity. 'The idea that identity changes over time ... remains stubbornly underdeveloped in so-called high theory', she complains.[9] Identity theorists (like eighteenth-century historians) have concentrated on imposed, internalized subject positions, and treat identity as 'being in a permanent fix'.[10]

She points to the fact that identities are not static, but made and re-made over time, suggesting that it is possible to have 'multiple selves' sequentially: something not unlike the ideas encountered in my exposition in this book. Gullette stresses the performative nature of aging, describing the concept of age identity as potential for 'a series of try-ons and reaffirmed performances'.[11] She sets out her vision for a new vision of age-informed identity:

> I think that identity over time can be seen as a sense of an achieved portmanteau 'me' – made up, for each subject, of all its changeable and continuing selves together – connected in different ways, or intermittently, but sometimes barely at all, to a sensuously material body'.[12]

It cannot have escaped notice that some of the desirables that Gullette sees in a vibrantly post-modern vision of aging identity were in fact present in the eighteenth-century imagination. It seems entirely possible that many eighteenth-century writers would have considered themselves 'aged by culture', although they would not of course have expressed it in such terms.

Finding out about how our eighteenth-century forebears made sense of aging can be a way to access underlying structures of epoch specific thought: not only about the physical body, but also about the nature of selfhood, the limits of nature and culture, choice and destiny. Adding age and aging to the historian's toolkit forces us to acknowledge the historical specificity of our own foundational categories – in the way that we now take for granted about class, race and gender. Contemporary social theorists and Gerontologists might be surprised to learn that their apparently progressive, liberating visions are not in fact new but actually reflect how we used to think about age and identity several centuries ago. This brings us full-circle: to the point with which I started this book. History won't help us solve the problems we face in our own aging society, but it does show us what is so historical about the problems we face and the questions we ask. In time, contemporary theorists may come to benefit from a perspective informed by historical analysis of age and aging.

NOTES

Introduction

1. R. Martin and J. Barresi, *Naturalization of the Soul: Self and Personal Identity in the Eighteenth Century* (London, 2000), p. ix.
2. J. Locke, *Essay Concerning Human Understanding* (London, 1690), I.4.4.
3. R. Atchley, *Social Forces and Aging: An Introduction to Social Gerontology* (Belmont, CA, 2000), p. 526.
4. D. Kertzner and J. Keith (eds), *Age and Anthropological Theory* (Ithaca, NY and London: Cornell University Press, 1984); Atchley, *Social Forces and Aging*; A. Bowling et al. (eds), 'Attributes of Age-identity', *Ageing & Society*, 25 (2005), pp. 479–500; G. Kaufman and G. Elder 'Revisiting Age Identity: A Research Note', *Journal of Aging Studies*, 16:2 (May 2002), pp. 169–76; S. Munson Deats and L. Tallent Lenker (eds), *Aging and Identity: A Humanities Perspective* (London: Greenwood Publishing Group, 1999); C. Ryff and V. W. Marshall (eds), *The Self and Society in Aging Processes* (New York: Springer Publishing Company, 1999).
5. M. M. Gullette, *Aged by Culture* (Chicago, IL: University of Chicago Press, 2004), p. 99.
6. S. Arber and J. Ginn (eds), *Connecting Gender & Ageing: A Sociological approach* (Buckingham, Philadelphia, PA: Open University Press, 1995), p. 5.
7. Kertzner and Keith (eds), *Age and Anthropological Theory*, p. 21.
8. K. Thomas, 'Age and Authority in Early Modern England', *Proceedings of the British Academy*, 62 (1976), pp. 205–48, on p. 205.
9. See D. G. Troyansky, 'Historical Research into Ageing, Old Age and Older People', in A. Jamieson, S. Harper and C. Victor (eds), *Critical Approaches to Ageing and Later Life* (Buckingham, Philadelphia, PA, 1997), pp. 49–62.
10. P. Laslett, *Family Life and Illicit Love in Earlier Generations: Essays in Historical Sociology* (Cambridge: Cambridge University Press, 1977), p. 181.
11. P. Laslett, 'The Significance of the Past in the Study of Ageing', *Ageing and Society*, 4:4 (1984), pp. 379–89.
12. P. Laslett, *A Fresh Map of Life: The Emergence of the Third Age* (London: Weidenfeld and Nicolson, 1989).
13. P. Thane, *Old Age in English History: Past Experiences, Present Issues* (Oxford: Oxford University Press, 2000), p. 1.
14. Ibid., p. 55–70.
15. S. Ottaway, *The Decline of Life: Old Age in Eighteenth-Century England* (Cambridge: Cambridge University Press, 2004), p. 278.
16. Ibid., pp. 12, 26, 45–52, 279.

17. L. Botelho, 'Old Age and Menopause in Rural Women of Early Modern Suffolk', in L .Botelho and P. Thane (eds), *Women and Aging in British Society since 1500* (London: Pearson Education, 2001), p.53.

18. Botelho and Thane (eds), *Women and Aging in British Society since 1500*, p. 3.

19. See K. Kitteridge, 'The Ag'd Dame to Venery Inclin'd: Images of Sexual Older Women in Eighteenth-Century Britain', in S. Ottaway, L. A. Botelho and K. Kitteridge, *Power and Poverty: Old Age in the Pre-Industrial Past* (London: Praeger, 2002), pp. 248–59; J. M. Casler, 'Aging and Opportunity: Growing Older in Clara Reeve's *School for Widows* (1791)', *Journal of Aging and Identity*, 4:2 (June 1999), pp. 291–310; L. Botelho, 'Images of Old Age in Early Modern Cheap Print: Women, Witches and the Poisonous Female Body', in *Power and Poverty: Old Age in the Pre-Industrial Past*, pp. 226–40; Botelho, 'Old Age and Menopause', pp. 52–69; A. C. L. Beam, '"Should I as Yet Call You Old?" Testing the Boundaries of Female Old Age in Early Modern England', in E. Campbell (ed.), *Growing Old in Early Modern Europe; Cultural Representations* (Aldershot and Burlington, VT: Ashgate Publishing Limited, 2006), pp. 98–114.

20. A. Kugler, '"I Feel Myself Decay Apace": Old Age in the Diary of Lady Sarah Cowper 1644–1720', in *Women and Aging in British Society since 1500*, pp. 70–85.

21. L. Botelho, 'When the Healer becomes the Patient: Old Age and Illness in the Life of Elizabeth Freke, 1641–1714', in C. Streubel (ed.), *Aging Stories: Narrative Constructions of Age and Gender* (Frankfurt and New York, 2009).

22. Ottaway, *The Decline of Life*, p. 6.

23. J. Gillis, *Youth and History: Tradition and Change in European Age Relations 1770–Present* (London: Academic Press, 1981), p. 39.

24. Ottaway, *The Decline of Life*, p. 7.

25. Ibid., p. 11.

26. Ibid., p. 12.

27. L. I. Conrad et al. (eds), *The Western Medical Tradition 800 BC to AD 1800* (Cambridge, 1995); K. Figlio, 'The Historiography of Scientific Medicine: An Invitation to the Human Sciences', *Comparative Studies in Society and History*, 19:3 (July 1977), pp. 262–86; C. Jones and R. Porter (eds), *Reassessing Foucault: Power, Medicine and the Body* (London and New York: Routledge, 1994).

28. See Chapter 3.

29. See M. Abbott, *Life Cycles in England 1560–1720: Cradle to Grave* (London and New York: Routledge, 1996), p.16.

30. See A. Wilson, 'The Politics of Medical Improvement in Early Hanoverian London', in A. Cunningham and R. French, *The Medical Enlightenment of the Eighteenth Century* (Cambridge: Cambridge University Press, 1990), pp. 4–39.

31. See L. E. Klein, 'Politeness and the Interpretation of the British Eighteenth Century', *Historical Journal*, 45:4 (2002), pp. 869–98; P. Langford, *A Polite and Commercial People, England 1727–1780* (Oxford: Oxford University Press, 1989), pp. 65, 91–2; Quote from L. E. Klein, *Shaftesbury and the Culture of Politeness: Moral Discourse and Cultural Politics in Early Eighteenth-Century England* (Cambridge: Cambridge University Press, 1994), p. 4.

32. R. Porter, 'Lay Medical Knowledge in the Eighteenth-Century: The Evidence of the *Gentleman's Magazine*', *Medical History*, 29:2 (1985), pp. 138–45.

33. G. Cheyne, *An Essay of Health and Long Life* (London, 1724), p. 1.

34. Ibid., p. xiv.

35. M. M. Roberts, 'A Physic against Death: Eternal Life and the Enlightenment – Gender and Gerontology', in M. M. Roberts and R. Porter (eds), *Literature and Medicine during the Eighteenth Century* (London: Routledge, 1993), pp. 151–67; G. S. Rousseau, 'Science Books and their Readers in the Eighteenth Century', in I. Rivers (ed.), *Books and their Readers in Eighteenth-Century England* (Leicester, 1982), p. 231.

36. L. Jordanova, *The Sense of a Past in Eighteenth-Century Medicine* (Reading: University of Reading, 1999), p. 6. See J. Black, *The English Press in the Eighteenth Century* (London: Taylor & Francis, 1987); J. A. Downie and T. N. Corns (eds), *Telling People What to Think: Early Eighteenth-Century Periodicals from the Review to the Rambler* (London, 1993); H. Barker, *Newspapers, Politics, and Public Opinion in Late Eighteenth-Century England* (Oxford: Clarendon Press, 1998); T. Feist, *The Stationer's Voice: The English Almanac Trade in the Early Eighteenth Century* (Philadelphia, PA: Amer Philosophical Society, 2005); C. Auf dem Keller, *Textual Structures in Eighteenth-Century Newspaper Advertising: a Corpus-Based Study of Medical Advertisements and Book Advertisements* (Aachen: Shaker Verlag GmbH, 2004).

37. Rousseau, 'Science books', p. 232.

38. R. Porter, 'The Eighteenth Century', in *The Western Medical Tradition*, p. 444.

39. T. Tryon, *The Way to Health, Long Life and Happiness* (London, 1691).

40. Dr. Trusler, *A Sure Way to Strengthen Life with Vigour: Particularly in Old Age; the Result of Experience* (London, 1819).

41. G. J. Gruman, 'A History of Ideas about the Prolongation of Life: The Evolution of Prolongevity Hypotheses to 1800', *Transactions of the American Philosophical Society*, 56:9 (1966), pp. 6–85, on p. 6.

42. D. B. Haycock, *This Mortal Coil: A Short History of Living Longer* (New Haven, CT and London: Yale University Press, 2008).

43. Roberts, 'A Physic against Death', p. 151.

44. Ibid., p. 164.

45. See J. G. Evans, 'Geriatric Medicine: A Brief History', *British Medical Journal*, 315 (1997), pp. 1075–77.

46. Mullan, *Sentiment and Sociability: The Language of Feeling in the Eighteenth Century* (Oxford: Clarendon Press, 1988), p. 203.

47. See A. Guerrini, *Obesity and Depression in the Enlightenment: the Life and Times of George Cheyne* (London: University of Oklahoma Press, 1999).

48. D. E. Shuttleton, '"Pamela's Library": Samuel Richardson and Dr. Cheyne's 'Universal Cure', *Eighteenth-Century Life*, 23:1 (1999), p. 61.

49. Rousseau, 'Science books', p. 217.

50. See G. S Rousseau, 'J. S. Hill, Universal Genius *Manqué*: Remarks on his Life and Times, with a Checklist of his Works', in J. A. L. Lemay and G. S. Rousseau (eds), *The Renaissance Man in the Eighteenth Century* (Los Angeles, CA, 1978), pp. 45–129.

51. P. Thicknesse, *The Valetudinarians Bath Guide: or, The Means of Obtaining Long Life and Health* (London, 1780), p.17.

52. See P. Otto, '"Performing the Resurrection": James Graham and the Multiplication of the Real', *Cultural and Social History*, 3:3 (2006), pp. 325–40; Quote from Roberts, 'A Physic against Death', p. 15.

53. Mullan, *Sentiment and Sociability*, p. 205.

54. Cheyne, *An Essay of Health*, p. 2; W. Buchan, *Domestic Medicine: or, The Family Physician* (London, 1769), pp. x–xi.

55. Buchan, *Domestic Medicine*, p. x.

56. This statement was included in the extended title of Buchan's work: *Domestic Medicine: or, The Family Physician: Being an Attempt to Render the Medical Art more Generally Useful, by Shewing People What is in their Own Power Both with Respect to the Prevention and Cure of Diseases.*

57. Porter, 'The Eighteenth Century', p. 445.

58. See A. Emch-Deriaz, 'The Non-naturals Made Easy', in Porter (ed.), *The Popularization of Medicine*, pp. 134–59.

59. B. Duden, 'Medicine and the History of the Body: The Lady of the Court', in J. Lachmund and G. Stollberg (eds), *The Social Construction of Illness: Illness and Medical Knowledge in Past and Present* (Stuttgart: Koch, Neff & Oetinger & Co, 1992), pp. 47–50.

60. See A. T. McKenzie, 'The Countenance You Show Me: Reading the Passions in the Eighteenth Century', *Georgia Review*, 32:4 (Winter 1978), pp. 758–73, on p. 759.

61. Descartes, R., *The Passions of the Soule in Three Books* (London, 1650), p. 24.

62. J. Monro, *Remarks on Dr. Battie's Treatise on Madness* (London, 1758), p. 45.

63. H. D. Gaubius, *On the Passions: or A Philosophical Discourse Concerning the Duty and Office of Physicians in the Management and Cure of the Disorders of the Mind* (London, 1760), p. 52.

64. Cheyne, *An Essay of Health*, p. 144.

65. Buchan, *Domestic Medicine*, p. 112.

1 Words and Concepts: The Meaning of Age and Aging

1. See: Ottaway, *The Decline of Life*, pp. 16–62; J. Roebuck, 'When Does Old Age Begin? The Evolution of the English Definition', *Journal of Social History*, 12:3 (Spring 1979), pp. 416–29; M. Dove, *The Perfect Age of Man's Life* (Cambridge: Cambridge University Press, 1986), pp. 37–45; Thane, *Old Age in English History*; Abbott, *Life Cycles in England*; Laslett, *Family Life and Illicit Love in Earlier Generations*, pp. 174–213; T. K. Hareven, 'The Life Course and Aging in Historical Perspective', in T. K. Hareven and K. J. Adams (eds), *Ageing and Life Course Transitions: An Interdisciplinary Perspective* (London and New York: Routledge, 1982), pp. 1–26.; Troyansky, 'Historical Research into Ageing', pp. 49–62.

2. Ottaway, *The Decline of Life*, p. 44.

3. In this respect I am indebted to Naomi Tadmor, who outlined this approach in her article, 'The Concept of the Household-Family in Eighteenth-Century England', *Past and Present*, 151 (May 1996), pp. 111–40, on p. 133.

4. 'Historical epistemology' has been defined by L. Daston as 'the history of the categories that structure our thought, pattern our arguments and proofs, and certify our standards of explanation'. L. Daston, 'Historical Epistemology', in J. Chandler et al. (eds), *Questions of Evidence: Proof, Practice, and Persuasion across the Disciplines* (Chicago, IL: University of Chicago Press Journals, 1994). 'Unstructured institutions' comes from D. Wahrman, *The Making of the Modern Self* (New Haven, CT and London, 2004), p. xv.

5. B. Lynch, *A Guide to Health through the Various Stages of Life* (London, 1744), p. 16.

6. J. Hill, *The Old Man's Guide to Health and Longer Life* (London, 1764), p. 4.

7. J. Hill, *The Virtues of Sage, in Lengthening Human Life: With Rules to Attain Old Age in Health and Cheerfulness* (London, 1765), p. 10.

8. J. Bethum, *A Short View of the Human Faculties and Passions* (Edinburgh, 1770), p. 113.

9. E. Chambers and A. Rees, *Cyclopædia: or, An Universal Dictionary of Arts and Sciences* (London, 1728; 1778–88), c.f. 'age'.

10. Dove, *The Perfect Age of Man's Life*, p. 12.
11. R. Samber, *Long Livers: A Curious History of Such Persons of Both Sexes who have Liv'd Several Ages, and Grown Young Again* (London, 1722).
12. See 'The Life Cycle' in Chapter 2.
13. Chambers and Rees, *Cyclopædia*, c.f. 'age'.
14. Dove, *The Perfect Age of Man's Life*, pp. 10–20.
15. E. Maynwaringe, *The Method and Means of Enjoying Health, Vigour, and Long Life* (London, 1683), p. 25.
16. Ibid., p. iv.
17. J. Taylor, *Annals of Health and Long Life* (London, 1818), p. 91.
18. Samber, *Long Livers*, p. 42.
19. R. Browne (trans.), *The Cure of Old Age, and Preservation of Youth, by Roger Bacon* (London, 1683), p. ii.
20. Ibid., p. 23
21. Ibid., p. 2.
22. Ibid., p. 95.
23. R. Steele, *A Discourse Concerning Old-Age: Tending to the Instruction, Caution and Comfort of Aged Persons* (London, 1688), p. 1.
24. Ibid., p. 5.
25. Ibid., p. 6.
26. Ibid., p.7.
27. Ibid., pp.7–8.
28. Ibid., pp. 9–10.
29. E. Wilson (trans.), *Hufeland's Art of Prolonging Life* (London, 1853), p. xi.
30. Ibid., p. 176.
31. Ibid., p. 176.
32. S. Clark, 'Inversion, Misrule and the Meaning of Witchcraft', *Past and Present*, 87 (May 1980), pp. 98–127; S. Clark, *Thinking with Demons: The Idea of Witchcraft in Early Modern Europe* (Oxford, 1997).
33. Clark, *Thinking with Demons*, p. 105.
34. See K. M. Davies, 'Continuity and Change in Literary Advice on Marriage', in R. B. Outhwaite (ed.), *Marriage and Society: Studies in the Social History of Marriage* (London: Europa, 1981), pp. 58–80; Botelho, 'Images of Old Age in Early Modern Cheap Print', pp. 217–36; K. Shevelow, *Women and Print Culture: The Construction of Femininity in the Early Periodical* (London and New York: Taylor & Francis, 1989); N. Armstrong and L. Tennenhouse (eds), *The Ideology of Conduct: Essays on Literature and the History of Sexuality* (New York and London: Routledge, 1987), pp. 1–25; C. H. Flynn, 'Defoe's Idea of Conduct: Ideological Fictions and Fictional Reality', in N. Armstrong and L. Tennenhouse (eds), *The Ideology of Conduct*, pp. 73–95; Kitteridge, 'The Ag'd Dame to Venery Inclin'd:'.
35. D. Defoe, *Conjugal Lewdness: or Matrimonial Whoredom* (London, 1727), p. 230.
36. Davies, 'Continuity and Change in Literary Advice on Marriage', p. 65.
37. H. Swinburne, *A Treatise of Spousals, or Matrimonial Contracts* (London, 1711), p. 47.
38. Thomas, 'Age and Authority in Early Modern England', p. 244.
39. See I. K. Ben-Amos, *Adolescence and Youth in Early Modern England* (New Haven, CT and London: Yale University Press, 1994), pp. 10–38; Thane, *Old Age in English History*, pp. 55–70; Ottaway, *The Decline of Life*, p. 32; L. Gowing, *Common Bodies: Women,*

Touch & Power in Seventeenth-Century England (Oxford: Yale University Press, 2003), pp. 15, 22, 47.

40. G. Booth, *The Present State of Matrimony: or, The Real Causes of Conjugal Infidelity and Unhappy Marriages* (London, 1739), pp. 32–3.

41. P. Stallybrass and A. White, *The Politics and Poetics of Transgression* (London: Taylor & Francis, 1986), p. 23.

42. Tryon, *The Way to Health*, p. 454.

43. *The Batchelor's Monitor: With Healthy and Pleasant Advice for Married Men in the Governing a Wife: To which is added, An Essay against Unequal Marriages* (London, 1743), p. 145.

44. S. L. Gilman, *Difference and Pathology: Stereotypes of Sexuality, Race, and Madness* (Ithaca, NY and London: Cornell University Press, 1985), pp. 15–37.

45. T. Castle, *Masquerade and Civilization: The Carnivalesque in Eighteenth-Century English Culture and Fiction* (Stanford, CA: Stanford University Press, 1986), p. 5.

46. E. Ward, *The Amorous Bugbears: or, The Humours of a Masquerade* (London, 1725), pp. 21–2.

47. B. Marshall, 'Science, Medicine and Virility Surveillance: The New Biology of "Sexy Seniors"', paper presented at *(Re)constructing the Aging Body: Western Medical Cultures and Gender 1600–2000*, Mainz, Germany, 26–8 September 2008.

48. Laslett, *Family Life and Illicit Love in Earlier Generations*, p. 181.

2 The Forces of Aging: Macrocosm and Microcosm

1. N. L. Stepan, 'Race, Gender, Science and Citizenship', *Gender and History*, 10 (1998), p. 29.

2. See T. Laqueur, *Making Sex: Body and Gender from the Greeks to Freud* (Cambridge, MA and London: Harvard University Press, 1990); G. J. Barker-Benfield, *The Culture of Sensibility: Sex and Society in Eighteenth-Century Britain* (London and Chicago, IL: University of Chicago Press, 1992); C. Gallagher and T. Laqueur (eds), *The Making of the Modern Body: Sexuality and Society in the Nineteenth Century* (Berkeley, Los Angeles, CA and London: University of California Press, 1987); A. Fletcher, *Gender, Sex, and Subordination in England 1500–1800* (New Haven, CT and London: Yale University Press, 1995); R. B. Shoemaker, *Gender in English Society, 1650–1850: the Emergence of Separate Spheres?* (London: Longman, 1998); T. Hitchcock, *English Sexualities, 1700–1800* (London: Palgrave Macmillan, 1997); R. Porter, *Flesh in the Age of Reason: How the Enlightenment Transformed the Way We See Our Bodies and Souls* (London: W. W. Norton & Co., 2003); K. Harvey, 'The Substance of Sexual Difference: Change and Persistence in Representations of the Body in c18 England', *Gender & History*, 14:2 (August 2002), pp. 202–23.

3. Laqueur, *Making Sex*, p. 154.

4. Ibid., p. 155.

5. Duden, 'Medicine and the History of the Body', p. 40.

6. Ottaway, *The Decline of Life*, p. 279.

7. Gowing, *Common Bodies*, p. 15.

8. R. Ralley, 'Climacterical Years: Astrology and Ageing in Early Modern England', paper presented at the Early Modern Philosophy and the Scientific Imagination seminar, London, 19 June 2009.

9. T. Browne, *Pseudodoxia epidemica*; quoted by Ralley, 'Climacterical Years'.

10. Ibid.

11. J. Partridge, *Defectio geniturarum, Being an Essay Toward the Reviving and Proving the True Old Principles of Astrology Hitherto Neglected or at Leastwise not Observed or Understood* (London, 1697), p. 90.

12. M. Stolberg, 'Female Menopause and Male Climacteric in Pre-modern Medicine', paper presented at *(Re)constructing the Aging Body: Western Medical Cultures and Gender 1600–2000*, Mainz, Germany, 26–8 September 2008.

13. W. Massey (trans.), *Tully's Compendious Treatise of Old Age: Intitled Cato Major* (London, 1753), pp. vi–vii.

14. J. Taylor, 'The Old, Old, Very Old Man: or The Age and Long Life of Thomas Parr', in *Caulfield's Edition of Curious Tracts* (London, 1635: London, 1794), p. 9.

15. Lynch, *A Guide to Health*, pp. 1–2.

16. E. Strother, *The Family Companion for Health* (London, 1729), pp. 48–9.

17. Ibid., p. 49.

18. H. Boerhaave, *Dr. Boerhaave's Academical Lectures on the Theory of Physic* (London, 1742–6), vol. 3, p. 409.

19. Cheyne, *An Essay of Health*, p. 295.

20. Lynch, *A Guide to Health*, p. 4.

21. Thane, *Old Age in English History*, p. 6.

22. J. H. Cohausen, *Hermippus Redidivus: or The Sage's Triumph over Old Age and the Grave* (London, 1743), p. 12.

23. Steele, *A Discourse Concerning Old-Age*, p. 5.

24. Ibid., pp. 12–20.

25. J. Harris, *The Divine Physician: Prescribing Rules for the Prevention, and Cure of Most Diseases as well of the Body, as the Soul* (Norwich, 1709), pp. 22, 165.

26. Shuttleton, '"Pamela's Library": Samuel Richardson and Dr. Cheyne's "Universal Cure"', *Eighteenth-Century Life*, 23:1 (1999), pp. 59–79, on pp. 60–1.

27. Cheyne, *An Essay of Health*, p. 206.

28. Shuttleton, 'Pamela's Library', p. 60.

29. J. Wesley, *Primitive Physick: or, An Easy and Natural Method of Curing Most Diseases* (London, 1747), p. xv.

30. Ibid., p. iii.

31. S. Aynscough, *A General Index to the First Fifty-six Volumes of the Gentleman's Magazine, from its Commencement in the Year 1731 to the End of 1786* (London, 1789). c.f. Age, remarkable instances of.

32. Taylor, 'The Old, Old, Very Old Man'.

33. See R. Willis (trans.), 'The Anatomical Examination of the body of Thomas Parr', in *The Works of William Harvey, M.D, Physician to the King, Professor of Anatomy and Surgery to the College of Physicians* (London, 1847), pp. 589–92.

34. Thomas, 'Age and Authority in Early Modern England', p. 61.

35. Cohausen, *Hermippus Redidivus*, p. 6.

36. Ibid., p. 6.

37. Ibid., p. 12.

38. Barker-Benfield, *The Culture of Sensibility*, p. 3.

39. Browne (trans.), *The Cure of Old Age, and Preservation of Youth*, p. 23.

40. Cheyne, *An Essay of Health*, p. 226.

41. Cohausen, *Hermippus Redidivus*, p. 11; Wilson, *Hufeland's Art of Prolonging Life*.

42. Duden, 'Medicine and the History of the Body', pp. 39–52; S. Pilloud and M. Louis-Courvoisier, 'The Intimate Experience of the Body in the Eighteenth Century: Between

Interiority and Exteriority' *Medical History*, 47 (October 2003), pp. 451–72; P. Rieder, 'Patients and Words: a Lay Medical Culture?', in G. S. Rousseau, M. Gill, D. Boyd Haycock and M. Herwig (eds), *Framing and Imagining Disease in Cultural History* (Basingstoke: Palgrave Macmillan, 2003), pp. 215–26.

43. 'Eminent Physician', *The Nurse's Guide ... To which is Added, an Essay on Preserving Health, and Prolonging Life* (London, 1729), p. 81.

44. J. Floyer, *Medicina gerocomica: or, the Galenic art of Preserving Old Men's Healths* (London, 1724), p. xvi.

45. Monro, *Remarks on Dr. Battie's Treatise*, pp. 26–7.

46. Lynch, *A Guide to Health*, p. 1.

47. W. Cullen (trans.) *Haller's First Lines of Physiology* (Edinburgh, 1786), p. 85.

48. Lynch, *A Guide to Health*, pp. 1–2.

49. Bethum, *A Short View of the Human Faculties*, pp. 82, 113.

50. This was the title of Lynch's first chapter in *A Guide to Health through the Various Stages of Life* (1744).

51. Bethum, A *Short View of the Human Faculties*, p. 82.

52. Gaubius, *On the Passions*, p. 88.

53. R. Paulson, 'Life as a Journey and as Theater: Two Eighteenth-Century Narrative Structures', *New Literary History*, 8:1 (Autumn 1976), pp. 43–58; D. Marshall, 'Adam Smith and the Theatricality of Moral Sentiments', *Critical Inquiry*, 10:4 (June 1984), pp. 593–4.

54. Steele, *A Discourse on Old-Age*, p. 10.

55. Strother, *Family Companion*, p. 50.

56. 'True Penitent', *The Folly, Sin, and Danger of Marrying Widows, and Old Women in General, Demonstrated And Earnestly Address'd to the Batchelors of Great Britain* (London, 1746), p. 29.

57. Lynch, *A Guide to Health*, p. 7.

58. 'Eminent Physician', *The Nurse's Guide*, p. 81.

59. Steele, *A Discourse Concerning Old-Age*, p. 1.

60. Cheyne, *An Essay of Health*, preface.

61. W. Temple, 'Of Health and Long Life', *The Works of Sir William Temple* (London, 1710), vol. 1, pp. 272–90, on p. 275.

62. Cheyne, *An Essay of Health*, p. 226; Buchan, *Domestic Medicine*, p. xii.

63. Quoted in R. Porter, *Bodies Politic: Disease, Death and Doctors in Britain, 1650–1900* (Ithaca, NY: Cornell University Press, 2001), p. 60.

64. Cheyne, *An Essay of Health*, p. 220.

65. Floyer, *Medicina gerocomica*, p. 10.

66. Ibid., p. 4.

67. Duden, 'Medicine and the History of the Body', p. 49.

68. Floyer, *Medicina gerocomica*, p. 10.

69. Ibid., p.10.

70. Ibid., p. 4.

71. J. Floyer, *The Ancient Psychrolousia Revived, or, An Essay to Prove Cold Bathing both Safe and Useful* (London, 1702).

72. Ibid.

73. Floyer, *Medicina gerocomica*, p. 6.

74. Porter, 'The Eighteenth Century' p. 415.

75. A. Wear, 'Medicine in Early Modern Europe, 1500–1700', in Conrad et al. (eds), *The Western Medical Tradition*, p. 360.

3 The New Science: Aging and Agency

1. See S. Jacyna, 'Medicine in Transformation, 1800–1849', in Conrad et al. (eds), *The Western Medical Tradition*, pp. 11–101; G. S. Rousseau et al., *Framing and Imagining Disease in Cultural History* (Basingstoke: Palgrave Macmillan, 2003); Barker-Benfield, *The Culture of Sensibility*; A. Cunningham and R. French (eds), *The Medical Enlightenment of the Eighteenth Century*; R. Smith, *Fontana History of the Human Sciences* (London: Fontana Press, 1997), Part III: 'The Long Eighteenth Century'; Wear, 'Medicine in Early Modern Europe', pp. 215–370; P. Goring, *The Rhetoric of Sensibility in Eighteenth-Century Culture* (Cambridge: Cambridge University Press, 2005); Mullan, *Sentiment and Sociability*; G. S. Rousseau, 'Nerves, Spirits, and Fibres: Towards Defining the Origins of Sensibility', in R. F. Brissenden and J. C. Eade (eds), *Studies in the Eighteenth Century III* (Toronto and Buffalo: University of Toronto Press, 1976), pp. 137–58; G. S. Rousseau (ed.), *The Languages of Psyche: Mind and Body in Enlightenment Thought* (Berkeley, Los Angeles, CA and London, 1990).
2. D. Schafer, *Old Age and Disease in Early Modern Medicine* (London: Pickering & Chatto, 2011).
3. 'Newtonising' quoted in Porter, 'The Eighteenth Century', p. 415. 'Deontologizing of the world of matter' quoted in P. Otto, 'Performing the Resurrection', p. 328.
4. Descartes, *The Passions of the Soule*, p. 4.
5. Barker-Benfield, *The Culture of Sensibility*, p. xvii.
6. Cunningham, *The Medical Enlightenment of the Eighteenth Century*, pp. 40–66.
7. J. Browne (trans.), *Boerhaave's Institutions in Physick* (London, 1715), p. 9.
8. Boerhaave, *Dr. Boerhaave's Academical Lectures*, vol. 3, p. 342.
9. Ibid., vol. 3, p. 409.
10. Ibid., vol. 3, pp. 340–2.
11. J. Browne, *Boerhaave's Institutions*, pp. 317–8.
12. Ibid., pp. 317–8.
13. Boerhaave, *Dr. Boerhaave's Academical Lectures*, vol. 3, p. 409.
14. Ibid., vol. 3, p. 409.
15. Ibid., vol. 3, pp. 340–2.
16. See M. W. Riley (ed.), *Aging from Birth to Death: Interdisciplinary Perspectives* (Boudler: Westview Press, 1979), pp. 4–5.
17. Boerhaave, *Dr. Boerhaave's Academical Lectures*, vol. 3, p. 342.
18. Porter, 'The Eighteenth Century', p. 397.
19. Wear, 'Medicine in Early Modern Europe', p. 375.
20. Mullan, *Sentiment and Sociability*, p. 232.
21. Cullen, *Haller's First Lines of Physiology*, vol. 2, p. 239.
22. Ibid., vol. 2, p. 244.
23. Ibid., vol. 2, pp. 242–3.
24. Ibid., vol. 2, p. 242.
25. Ibid., vol. 2, pp. 241–2.
26. Ibid., vol. 2, p. 244.
27. Boerhaave, *Dr. Boerhaave's Academical Lectures*, vol. 3, p. 342.
28. Ibid., vol. 3, p. 342.
29. Cullen, *Haller's First Lines of Physiology*, vol. 2, p. 242.
30. J. Delacoste (trans.), *Boerhaave's Aphorisms* (London, 1715), p. 15.
31. Boerhaave, *Dr. Boerhaave's Academical Lectures*, vol. 3, p. 409.

32. Ibid, vol. 3, p. 409.

33. Cullen, *Haller's First Lines of Physiology*, vol. 2, p. 247.

34. E. Strother, *An Essay on Sickness and Health* (London, 1725), p. 1.

35. G. Cheyne, *The Natural Method of Cureing the Diseases of the Body, and the Disorders of the Mind Depending on the Body* (London, 1742), p. 295.

36. Ibid., p. 295.

37. Cheyne, *An Essay of Health*, p. 220.

38. Ibid., p. 220.

39. Cheyne, *The Natural Method*, pp. 293–4.

40. Ibid, p. 294.

41. Cheyne, *An Essay of Health*, p. 2.

42. Hill, *The Virtues of Sage*, p. 7.

43. Ibid., pp. 8–9.

44. Ibid., p. 8.

45. Ibid.

46. Ibid., p. 9.

47. Ibid., p. 7.

48. Ibid., p. 10.

49. J. Hill, *The Actor: A Treatise on the Art of Playing* (London, 1750).

50. Buchan, *Domestic Medicine*, pp. 48–50.

51. Ibid., p. 84.

52. G. Cheyne, *The English Malady: or A Treatise of Nervous Diseases of All Kinds* (London, 1733), p. 181.

53. Buchan, *Domestic Medicine*, p.145.

54. Monro, *Remarks on Dr. Battie's Treatise*, p. 27.

55. Cheyne, *An Essay of Health*, pp. 159–60.

56. See S. Foote, *A Treatise on the Passions, so far as they Regard the Stage* (London, 1747), pp. 8, 11; R. Pickering, *Reflections upon Theatrical Expression in Tragedy* (London, 1755), p. 17; J. Pittard, *Observations on Mr. Garrick's Acting* (London, 1758), p. 24; S. Derrick, *A General View of the Stage* (London, 1759), p. 92; W. Cooke, *The Elements of Dramatic Criticism* (London: Printed for G. Kearsly, 1775); W. Cooke, *The Life and Death of David Garrick, Esq.* (London, 1779), p. 13; T. Davies, *Memoirs of the Life of David Garrick* (London, 1780), pp. 77–9, 377–9.

57. Cheyne, *An Essay of Health*, pp. 159–60.

58. Ibid., p. 160.

59. Pickering, *Reflections upon Theatrical Expression in Tragedy*, p. 17.

60. Porter, 'The Character of an excellent Actor', *Gentleman's Magazine*, 13 (May 1743), pp. 253–5, on p. 255.

61. Foote, *A Treatise on the Passions*, p. 8.

62. J. Boswell, *The Life of Johnson* (Dublin, 1792), pp. vi, 66.

63. Barker-Benfield, *The Culture of Sensibility*, p. xvii.

64. Floyer, *Medicina gerocomica*, p. vii.

65. J. Floyer, *The Physician's Pulse Watch* (London, 1707–10), vol. 1, p. 23.

4 Society and Sociability: Cheerfulness

1. See J. Brewer, *The Pleasures of the Imagination: English Culture in the Eighteenth Century* (London: Farrar, Straus and Giroux, 1997); Jacyna, 'Medicine in transformation', pp. 11–101; Rousseau et al. (eds), *Framing and Imagining Disease in Cultural History*; Barker-Benfield, *The Culture of Sensibility*; A. Goodden (ed.), *The Eighteenth Century Body: Art History, Literature, Medicine* (London: Peter Lang, 2002); Goring, *The Rhetoric of Sensibility*; McKenzie, 'The Countenance You Show Me', pp. 758–73; Mullan, *Sentiment and Sociability*; W. M. Reddy, *The Navigation of Feeling: A Framework for the History of Emotions* (Cambridge: Cambridge University Press, 2001); Rousseau (ed.), *The Languages of Psyche*, pp. 3–44; Rousseau, 'Nerves, Spirits, and Fibres', pp. 137–58.

2. Goring, *The Rhetoric of Sensibility*, p. ix.

3. McKenzie, 'The Countenance You Show Me', p. 762.

4. R. Brosch, 'Spectacular Emotions: Edmund Burke's Redefinition of Visible Identity', in Gobel et al. (eds), *Engendering Images of Man in the Long Eighteenth Century* (Trier: WVT Wissenschaftlicher Verlag, 2001), pp. 23–4.

5. J. R. Roach, *The Player's Passion: Studies in the Science of Acting* (Newark, London and Toronto: University of Delaware Press, 1985), p. 97.

6. Mullan, *Sentiment and Sociability*, p. 203.

7. R. Markley, 'Sentimentality as Performance: Shaftesbury, Sterne, and the Theatrics of Virtue', in F. Nussbaum and L. Brown *The New Eighteenth Century* (New York and London: Routledge, 1987), pp. 210–30, on p. 219.

8. Ibid., pp. 219–20.

9. Reddy, *The Navigation of Feeling*, p. xii.

10. S. Johnson, *A Dictionary of the English Language* (London, 1755), c.f. 'cheerful'.

11. W. Godwin, *An Enquiry Concerning Political Justice, and its Influence on General Virtue and Happiness* (Dublin, 1793), p. 399.

12. The original article 'Cheerfulness' appeared in *The Spectator*, p. 381. The version quoted here appeared in J. Addison, *Maxims, Observations, and Reflections, Moral, Political, and Divine* (London, 1720), pp. 93–104.

13. Addison, 'Cheerfulness', p. 94.

14. W. Charleton, *A Natural History of the Passions* (London, 1701), pp. 68–9.

15. Godwin, *An Enquiry Concerning Political Justice*, p. 338.

16. Addison, 'Cheerfulness', p. 101.

17. Ibid., p. 101.

18. Quoted in Floyer, *Medicina gerocomica*, p. 21.

19. R. Lucas, *An enquiry after Happiness* (London, 1734), vol. I p. 140.

20. Ibid., vol. 1, p. 140.

21. Ibid., vol. 1, p. 139.

22. *World*, 16 April 1790; *Sun*, 28 September 1793. The advertisement also appeared in several other numbers of *World*, *Oracle*, *Public Advertiser*, *Courier* and the *Evening Gazette* throughout 1793 and 1794.

23. *World*, 22 November 1791. This advertisement appeared ninety-five times in the *Observer*, *Star*, *Gazetteer* and *New Daily Advertiser*.

24. *Oracle*, 12 July 1799.

25. *New Daily Advertiser*, 9 June 1799.

26. Hill, *The Old Man's Guide*, p. 4.

27. Cheyne, *The Natural Method*, p. 228.

28. Bethum, A *Short View of the Human Faculties and Passions*, p. 51.
29. Addison, 'Cheerfulness', p. 92.
30. Ibid., p. 93.
31. L. Sterne, 'On Chearfulness', in *The Works of Laurence Sterne* (Dublin, 1774), vol. 6, p. 54.
32. Ibid., vol. 6, p. 55.
33. Addison, 'On Cheerfulness', p. 95.
34. Ibid., p. 93.
35. Rieder, 'Patients and Words', p. 219.
36. Cheyne, *An Essay of Health*, p. 171.
37. Buchan, *Domestic Medicine*, p. 23.
38. T. Beddoes, *A Lecture Introductory to a Course of Popular Instruction on the Constitution and Management of the Human Body* (Bristol, 1797), p. 27.
39. Floyer, *Medicina gerocomica*, p. 5.
40. Ibid., p. 21.
41. Ibid.
42. Descartes, *The Passions of the Soule*, p. 78.
43. *The Best and Easiest Method of Preserving Uninterrupted Health to Extreme Old Age* (London, 1748), pp. 189–90.
44. Hill, *The Old Man's Guide*, p. 4.
45. Ibid., p. 26.
46. Lucas, *An Enquiry After Happiness*, p. 140.
47. Addison, 'Cheerfulness', p. 101.
48. Delacoste, *Boerhaave's Aphorisms*, p. 284.
49. Cullen, *Haller's First Lines of Physiology*, vol. 2, p. 247.
50. Buchan, *Domestic Medicine*, p. 145.
51. Ibid., p. 146.
52. Ibid.
53. Lucas, *An Enquiry After Happiness*, pp. 139–40.
54. Cohausen, *Hermippus Redivivus*, p. 111.
55. Boswell, *The Life of Johnson*, pt. vii, Aetat 68.
56. Cheyne, *The English Malady*, pp. 181–2.
57. Ibid., pp. 181–2.
58. See Brewer, *The Pleasures of the Imagination*, pp. 88, 144, 196, 581–2, 610.
59. M. Akenside, 'Hymn to Cheerfulness', in M. Akensinde, *Odes on Several Subjects* (London, 1788), pp. 243–50.
60. Ibid., p. 243.
61. Ibid., p. 244.
62. Ibid.
63. Ibid., p. 245.
64. Godwin, *An Enquiry Concerning Political Justice*, p. 400.
65. Ibid., p. 394.
66. Ibid., p. 395.
67. Ibid., p. 397.
68. Cheyne, *The Natural Method*, p. 309.
69. 'Eminent Physician', *The Nurse's Guide*, p. 130.
70. Buchan, *Domestic Medicine*, p. 146.
71. Ibid., p. 119.
72. See Otto, 'Performing the Resurrection', pp. 325–40, on p. 328.

73. See Porter, *Flesh in the Age of Reason*, pp. 334–9; Martin and Barresi, *Naturalization of the Soul*, pp. 89–133; Marshall, 'Adam Smith and the Theatricality of Moral Sentiments', pp. 592–613; Wahrman, *Making of the Modern Self*, p. 174; L. Woods, *Garrick Claims the Stage: Acting as Social Emblem in Eighteenth-Century England* (Westport, CT and London: Greenwood Press, 1984), pp. 34–6; Mullan, *Sentiment and Sociability*; Markley, 'Sentimentality as Performance', pp. 210–12.
74. Cullen, *Haller's First Lines of Physiology*, p. 86.
75. Otto, 'Performing the Resurrection', p. 328.
76. W. Belcher, *Intellectual Electricity, Novum Organum of Vision, and Grand Mystic Secret* (London, 1798), preface.
77. Ibid., preface.
78. Ibid., p. iii.
79. Ibid., pp. ii–iii
80. J. Priestley, *Observations on Respiration, and the use of the Blood* (London, 1776), p. 3.
81. Beddoes, *A Lecture Introductory*, p. 27.
82. Porter, *Gentleman's Magazine*, 13 (May 1743), pp. 279–80; *Daily Gazetteer*, 20 May 1743.
83. Porter, *Gentleman's Magazine*, 13, p. 279; *Daily Gazeteer*, 20 May 1743.
84. Cohausen, *Hermippus Redidivus*, p. 11.
85. Ibid., p. 30.
86. Cheyne, *The Natural Method*, p. 303.
87. Addison, 'Cheerfulness', pp. 94–5.
88. Mullan, *Sentiment and Sociability*, p. 5.
89. Akenside, 'Hymn to Cheerfulness', p. 246.
90. Buchan, *Domestic Medicine*, p. 112.
91. Ibid., p. 112.
92. Boswell, *The Life of Johnson*, pt. viii, Aetat 70.
93. Thicknesse, *The Valetudinarians Bath Guide*, p. 22.

5 Ages Identities: Prescriptive Behaviour for 'Old Men'

1. Rousseau, 'Science books', p. 231.
2. Dr Trusler, *A Sure Way to Strengthen Life*, p. 167.
3. Hill, *The Old Man's Guide*, p. 3.
4. J. Fothergill, *Rules for the Preservation of Health* (London, 1762), p. 21.
5. T. Bernard, *Spurinna or the Comforts of Old Age* (London, 1816), p. 2.
6. Cheyne, *The English Malady*, p. 248.
7. Dr. Trusler, *A Sure Way to Strengthen Life*, p. iv.
8. *The Invalid: With the Obvious Means of Enjoying Health and Long Life* (London, 1804), p. vii.
9. R. W. Connell, *Masculinities* (Cambridge, 1995), p. 76–9.
10. Fletcher, *Gender, Sex and Subordination in England*; E. A. Foyster, *Manhood in Early Modern England: Honour, Sex and Marriage* (London and New York, 1999); A. Shepard, *Meanings of Manhood in Early Modern England* (Oxford: Oxford University Press, 2003); A. Shepard, 'From Anxious Patriarchs to Refined Gentlemen? Manhood in Britain, circa 1500–1700', *Journal of British Studies* 44 (April 2005), pp. 281–95; L. Davidoff and C. Hall, *Family Fortunes: Men and Women of the English Middle Class, 1780–1850* (Chicago, IL: University of Chicago Press, 1987); J. Tosh, 'Masculinities

in an Industrialising Society: Britain 1800–1914', *Journal of British Studies*, 44 (April 2005), pp. 330–42.

11. Klein, *Shaftesbury and the Culture of Politeness*, p. 8.
12. P. Carter, *Men and the Emergence of Polite Society, Britain 1660–1800* (London: Pearson Education, 2001), p. 31.
13. Fletcher, *Gender, Sex and Subordination*, p. 323.
14. Brewer, *The Pleasures of the Imagination*, p. 111.
15. M. Cohen, '"Manners" Make the Man: Politeness, Chivalry, and the Construction of Masculinity, 1750–1830', *Journal of British Studies*, 44 (April 2005), pp. 312–29, on p. 313.
16. T. Hitchcock and M. Cohen (eds), *English Masculinities 1660–1800* (London and New York: Longman, 1999), p. 2.
17. M. McCormack, *The Independent Man: Citizenship and Gender Politics in Georgian England* (Manchester: Manchester University Press, 2005).
18. Carter, 'James Boswell's Manliness', in Hitchcock and Cohen (eds), *English Masculinities*, pp. 111–30; H. French and M. Rothery, 'Upon your Entry into the World: Masculine Values and the Threshold of Adulthood among Landed Elites in England 1680–1800', *Social History*, 33:4 (November 2008), pp. 402–22.
19. Fletcher, *Gender, Sex and Subordination*, pp. 322–3.
20. Shepard, *Meanings of Manhood*, p. 9.
21. Massey (trans.), *Tully's Compendious Treatise*.
22. Browne (trans.), *The Cure of Old Age, and Preservation of Youth*, p. 23.
23. Carter, *Men and the Emergence of Polite Society*, p. 209.
24. Cheyne, *An Essay of Health*, p. 12.
25. Cheyne, *The Natural Method*, p. 309.
26. Cheyne, *An Essay of Health*, p. 49; Bernard, *Comforts of Old Age*, pp. 121–2.
27. *The Invalid*, p. 31.
28. Bernard, *Comforts of Old Age*, pp. 93–4
29. Thicknesse, *The Valetudinarians Bath Guide*, p.22.
30. Wilson, *Heufland's Art of Prolonging Life*, p. 325.
31. Bernard, *Comforts of Old Age*, pp. 91–3.
32. W. Nisbet, *The New Domestic Medicine* (London, 1809), p. xi.
33. Cohen, *Fashioning Masculinity*, p. 5.
34. Hill, *Old Man's Guide*, p. 33.
35. P. Carter, 'Men about Town: Representations of Foppery and Masculinity in Early Eighteenth-Century Urban Society', in H. Barker and E. Chalus (eds), *Gender in Eighteenth-Century England: Roles, Representations and Responsibilities* (London and New York: Longman, 1997), pp. 31–57.
36. Carter, *Men and the Emergence of Polite Society*, pp. 35–6, 59, 71; A. N. Walters, 'Conversation Pieces: Science and Politeness in Eighteenth-Century England', *History of Science*, 35:2:108 (June 1997), pp. 121–54.
37. Cheyne, *An Essay of Health*, p. vii.
38. Trusler, *Sure Means*, p. 138; Sinclair, *Code of Health and Longevity*, p. 79.
39. Buchan, *Domestic Medicine*, p. 145.
40. Ibid., p. 146.
41. Cheyne, *An Essay of Health*, p. 171.
42. J. Barrell, *The Birth of Pandora and the Division of Knowledge* (Basingstoke, 1992), pp. 63–88.

43. G. Cheyne, *Essay on Regimen*, p. xxxiv.

44. Ibid., p. 24.

45. Cheyne, *English Malady*, p. 127.

46. Hill, *Old Man's Guide*, p. 12.

47. Fothergill, *Rules*, p. 22.

48. J. Johnson, *The Economy of Health* (London, 1837), p. 216.

49. Ibid., p. 217.

50. Bernard, *Comforts of Old Age*, p. 64.

51. Ibid., p. 66.

52. K. Harvey, '"The Majesty of the Masculine-Form": Multiplicity and Male Bodies in Eighteenth Century Erotica', in *English Masculinities*, pp. 193–214.

53. Thicknesse, *The Valetudinarians Bath Guide*, p. 17.

54. Ibid., p. 15.

55. Ibid., p. 22.

56. McCormack, *The Independent Man*, p. 5.

57. Thicknesse, *The Valetudinarians Bath Guide*, p. 15.

58. Cheyne, *An Essay of Health*, p. 94.

59. R. Warner (ed.), *Original Letters* (Bath and London, 1817), p. 80.

60. Kugler, 'I Feel myself Decay Apace', p. 95.

61. Stepan, 'Race, Gender, Science and Citizenship', p. 29.

62. J. Gregory, '*Homo Religious*: Masculinity and Religion in the Long Eighteenth Century', in *English Masculinities*, pp. 85–110.

6 Identity Formations: Age and 'Character'

1. See Martin and Barresi, *Naturalization of the Soul*; C. Taylor, *Sources of the Self: The Making of Modern Identity* (Cambridge, 1989); M. Carrithers, S. Collins and S. Lukes (eds), *The Category of the Person: Anthropology, Philosophy, History* (Cambridge: Cambridge University Press, 1985); R. Porter (ed.), *Rewriting the Self: Histories from the Renaissance to the Present* (London: Psychology Press, 1997); Porter, *Flesh in the Age of Reason*; F. Nussbaum, *The Autobiographical Subject: Gender and Ideology in Eighteenth-Century England* (Baltimore, MD and London, 1989); Wahrman, *Making of the Modern Self*; L. A. Freeman, *Character's Theater: Genre and Identity on the Eighteenth-Century English Stage* (Philadelphia, PA, 2002); Rousseau, *The Languages of Psyche*, pp. 3–44; D. S. Lynch, *The Economy of Character: Novels, Market Culture, and the Business of Inner Meaning* (Chicago, IL: University of Chicago Press, 1998).

2. Nussbaum, *The Autobiographical Subject*, pp. 38–9.

3. Wahrman, *Making of the Modern Self*, p. xi.

4. Porter, 'Introduction', in *Rewriting the Self*, pp. 1–17; p. 1.

5. Taylor, 'The Person', p. 258.

6. Mauss's essay was first given in his native French in 1938 at the Huxley Memorial Lecture, and consequently appeared in the *Journal of the Royal Anthropological Institute* 68 (1938). A translation by W. D. Halls, 'A Category of the Human Mind: The Notion of Person: the Notion of Self', appears in *The Category of the Person: Anthropology, Philosophy, History*, ed. M. Carrithers, S. Collins and S. Lukes (Cambridge: Cambridge University Press, 1985), pp. 1–25. The translation by W. D. Halls was commissioned for this volume with the permission of Routledge and Kegan Paul plc.

7. Mauss, 'A Category of the Human Mind: the Notion of Person: the Notion of Self', trans. Halls, in *The Category of the Person: Anthropology, Philosophy, History*, ed. Carrithers, Collins and Lukes, p. 20.
8. Mauss, 'A Category of the Human Mind', p. 22.
9. Ibid., p. 3.
10. Ibid.,p. 9.
11. Ibid., p. 14.
12. Ibid., p. 22.
13. Ibid., p. 22.
14. Porter, 'Introduction', in *Rewriting the Self*, p. 4.
15. For a specific discussion of Locke's definition of both the 'person' and the 'self', see Martin and Barresi, *Naturalization of the Soul*, pp. 20–1.
16. See Smith, *The Fontana History of The Human Sciences*, pp. 216–52. For Hartley and 'psychology' specifically, see p. 251.
17. Martin and Barresi, *Naturalization of the Soul*, p. ix.
18. Ibid., p. ix
19. Wahrman, *Making of The Modern Self*, p. 181.
20. I. Watt, *The Rise of the Novel* (Berkeley, CA: University of California Press, 1957). See Taylor, *Sources of the Self*, p. 287; Wahrman, *Making of the Modern Self*, p. 181; Nussbaum, *The Autobiographical Subject*; Lynch, *The Economy of Character*.
21. See Ottaway, *The Decline of Life*, pp. 16–62.
22. Ibid., p. 280.
23. M. Kohli, 'The World we Forgot: A Historical Review of the Life Course', in V. W. Marshall (ed.), *Later Life: The Social Psychology of Aging* (Beverly Hills, London, New Delhi: Sage, 1986), pp. 271–303.
24. Ibid., p. 284.
25. Kohli, 'The World We Forgot', pp. 271–303.
26. Wahrman, *Making of the Modern Self*, p. xvii.
27. Ibid., p. xiii.
28. See Nussbaum, 'Review of *The Making of the Modern Self*, by D. Wahrman, *The American Historical Review*, 110:3 (2005); Randall McGovern, 'Book Review of *The Making of the Modern Self*, by D. Wahrman', *Journal of British Studies*, 45:1 (2006), pp. 168–9; K. Berger, J. Campbell and D. Herzog, 'Book Review of *The Making of the Modern Self*, by D. Wahrman', *Eighteenth Century Studies*, 40:1 (2006), pp. 149–56.
29. Wahrman, *Making of the Modern Self*, p. xiii.
30. Ibid., p. 168.
31. S. Knott, 'A Cultural History of Sensibility in the Era of the American Revolution' (PhD dissertation, Oxford University, 1999), pp. 186–7. Quoted in Wahrman, *Making of the Modern Self*, p. 168.
32. See Lynch, *The Economy of* Character. The quote is from Porter, *Flesh in the Age of Reason*, p. 9.
33. Freeman, *Character's Theater*, pp. 11–46.
34. Ibid., p. 8.
35. Ibid., p. 39.
36. See pp. 128–36.
37. Smith, *The Fontana History of The Human Sciences*, p. 221.
38. Gaubius, *On the Passions*, p. 75.

39. Johnson, *A Dictionary of the English Language*, c.f. 'Character', 'person', 'quality', 'constitution', 'temperament', temper', 'manner', 'habit', 'condition', and 'complexion'.

40. Ibid., p. 91.

41. Ibid., p. 31–2.

42. Ibid., p. 90–1.

43. A. Downer, 'Nature to Advantage Dressed: Eighteenth-Century Acting' *Publications of the Modern Language Association of America*, 58:4:1 (December 1943), p. 1029; Roach, *The Player's Passion*, pp. 10–12.

44. E. Fischer-Lichte, 'Theatre and the Civilizing Process: An Approach to the History of Acting', in *Interpreting the Theatrical Past: Essays in the Historiography of Performance*, ed. T. Postlethwait and B. A. McConachie (Iowa: University of Iowa Press, 1989), pp. 34, 23.

45. P. Hiffernan, *Reflections on the Structure, and Passions of Man* (London, 1748); P. Hiffernan, *The Dramatic Genius* (London, 1770).

46. Hill, *The Actor*.

47. Ibid., p. 12.

48. Roach, *The Player's Passion*, p. 12.

49. Freeman, *Character's Theater*, pp. 6–7.

50. Goring, *Rhetoric of Sensibility*, p. 8.

51. Ibid., p. 7

52. C. Churchill, *The Rosciad* (London, 1761); R. Lloyd, *The Actor. A Poetical Epistle to Bonnell Thornton, Esq.* (London, 1760).

53. Ibid., pp. 8–9.

54. Downer, 'Nature to Advantage Dressed', p. 1027.

55. J. Boswell, 'On the Profession of a Player', *London Magazine, or Gentleman's Monthly Intelligencer*, 39 (1770) (August–October 1770); part I, August 1770, pp. 397–8; part II (September 1770), pp. 468–71. Essay III and last. (October 1770), pp. 513 – quote from part II, p. 468; Boswell, 'On the Profession of a Player', part II, p. 470.

56. Goring, *Rhetoric of Sensibility*, p. 128.

57. E. Curll, *The History of the English Stage, from the Restoration to the Present Time* (London, 1741), p. 48.

58. Ibid., pp. 49–50.

59. Ibid., p. 50.

60. D. Garrick, *An Essay on Acting* (London, 1744), pp. 9–10.

61. Porter, 'The Character of an Excellent Actor', p. 255.

62. Derrick, *A General View of the Stage*, p. 92.

63. Ibid., p. 92.

64. Thicknesse, *The Valetudinarians Bath Guide*, p. 23.

65. Paulson, 'Life as a Journey and as Theater', pp. 43–58.

66. Freeman, *Character's Theater*, p. 13

67. D. Marshall, *The Figure of Theater: Shaftesbury, Defoe, Adam Smith and George Eliot* (New York: Columbia University Press, 1986), pp. 4–5. Quoted in Freeman, *Character's Theater*, p. 13. See also J. C. Agnew, *Worlds Apart: The Market and the Theatre in Anglo-American Thought, 1550–1750* (Cambridge: Cambridge University Press, 1986).

68. Marshall, 'Adam Smith and the Theatricality of Moral Sentiments', pp. 593–4.

69. Ibid., p. 594.

70. J. Brewer, 'Commercialisation and Politics', in N. McKendrick, J. Brewer and J. H. Plumb, *The Birth of a Consumer Society: The Commercialisation of Eighteenth-Century England Society* (London, 1982), p. 213.

71. The quote is from Freeman, *Character's Theater*, p. 14.

72. A. Hill, 'The Distinction of Ages', in *The Works of the Late Aaron Hill* (London, 1754), vol. 4, p. 125.

73. Boswell, 'On the Profession of a Player', part I, p. 397.

74. Curll, *The History of the English Stage*, p. 48.

75. H. Fielding, *Tom Jones* (London, 1749), vol. 2, pp. vii, 174.

76. Freeman, *Character's Theater*, p. 7.

77. Martin and Barresi, *Naturalization of the Soul*, p. ix.

78. Figlio, 'The Historiography of Scientific Medicine', p. 285.

Conclusion

1. Ottaway, *The Decline of Life*, p. 45.

2. R. Poole, 'Give us our Eleven Days!' Calendar Reform in Eighteenth Century England' *Past and Present*, 149 (1995), pp. 95–139, on p. 96.

3. Cohausen, *Hermippus Redivivus*, p. 30.

4. Ibid., pp. 33–4

5. Porter, *Gentleman's Magazine*, p. 280.

6. S. Katz, 'A New Biopolitics of Age: Enhancement, Performance, Function', paper presented at *(Re)interpreting the Aging Body: Western Medical Cultures and Gender 1600–2000*, Mainz, Germany, 26–8 September 2008.

7. Gullette, 'Male Midlife Sexuality in a Gerontocratic Economy: The Privileged Stage of the Long Midlife in Nineteenth-Century Age Ideology', *Journal of the History of Sexuality*, 5:1 (July 1994), pp. 58–89 on p. 88.

8. Gullette, 'From Life Storytelling to Age Autobiography', *Journal of Aging Studies*, 18 (February 2003), pp. 101–11, on p. 101.

9. Gullette, *Aged by Culture*, p. 121.

10. Ibid., p. 122.

11. Ibid., p. 161.

12. Ibid., p. 125.

WORKS CITED

Primary Material

Addison, J., 'Chearfulness Preferable to Mirth', in J. Addison, *Maxims, Observations, and Reflections, Moral, Political, and Divine* (London, 1719–20).

Akenside, M., 'Ode VI: Hymn to Cheerfulness', in M. Akenside, *The Pleasures of the Imagination and Other Poems* (London, 1788), pp. 243–50.

—, 'The Pleasures of Imagination', in M. Akenside, *The Pleasures of the Imagination and Other Poems* (London, 1788).

Aynscough, S., *A General Index to the First Fifty-six Volumes of the Gentleman's Magazine, from its Commencement in the Year 1731 to the End of 1786* (London, 1786).

The Batchelor's Monitor: With Healthy and Pleasant Advice for Married Men in the Governing a Wife: To which is Added, An Essay against Unequal Marriages (London, 1743).

Beddoes, T., *A Lecture Introductory to a Course of Popular Instruction on the Constitution and Management of the Human Body* (Bristol, 1797).

Belcher, W., *Intellectual Electricity, Vobum Organum of Vision, and Grand Mystic Secret* (London, 1798).

Bernard, T., *Spurinna or the Comforts of Old Age* (London, 1816).

Bethum, J., *A Short View of the Human Faculties and Passions* (Edinburgh, 1770).

Boerhaave, H., *Dr. Boerhaave's Academical Lectures on the Theory of Physic* (London, 1742–6).

Booth, G., *The Present State of Matrimony: or, The Real Causes of Conjugal Infidelity and Unhappy Marriages* (London, 1739).

Boswell, J., 'On the Profession of a Player', *London Magazine, or Gentleman's Monthly Intelligencer*, 39 (1770), pp. 397–8, 468–71, 513.

—, *The Life of Samuel Johnson* (Dublin, 1792).

Brodum, W., *A Guide to Old Age, or A Cure for the Indiscretions of Youth* (London, 1795).

Browne, J. (trans.), *Boerhaave's Institutions in Physic* (London, 1715).

Browne, R. (trans.), *The Cure of Old Age, and Preservation of Youth, by Roger Bacon* (London, 1683).

Browne, T. *Pseudodoxia epidemica.*

Buchan, W., *Domestic Medicine; or, The Family Physician* (Edinburgh, 1769).

Byfield, T., *Directions Tending to Health and Long Life* (London, 1717).

Chambers, E, and A. Rees, *Cyclopædia: or, An Universal Dictionary of Arts and Sciences* (London, 1778–88).

—, *Cyclopædia: or, An Universal Dictionary of Arts and Sciences* (London, 1728).

'The Character of an Excellent Actor', *Gentleman's Magazine*, 13 (May 1743), p. 255.

Charleton, W., *A Natural History of the Passions* (London, 1701).

Cheyne, G., *An Essay on Regimen* (London, 1740).

—, *Dr. Cheyne's Own Account of Himself and of his Writings* (London, 1743).

—, *An Essay of Health and Long Life* (London, 1724).

—, *The English Malady: or, A Treatise of Nervous Diseases of All Kinds* (London, 1733).

—, *The Natural Method of Cureing the Diseases of the Body, and the Disorders of the Mind Depending on the Body* (London, 1742).

Churchill, C., *The Rosciad* (London, 1761).

Cohausen, J. H., *Hermippus Redivivus: or, The Sage's Triumph over Old Age and the Grave* (London, 1743).

Cullen, W. (trans.), *Haller's First Lines of Physiology* (Edinburgh, 1786).

Curll, E., *The History of the English Stage, from the Restoration to the Present Time* (London, 1741).

Defoe, D., *Conjugal Lewdness; or Matrimonial Whoredom* (London, 1727).

Delacoste, J. (trans.), *Boerhaave's Aphorisms: Concerning the Knowledge and Cure of Diseases* (London, 1715).

Derrick, S., *A General View of the Stage* (London, 1759).

Descartes, R., *The Passions of the Soule* (London, 1650).

Emch-Deriaz, A., 'The Non-naturals Made Easy', in Porter (ed.), *The Popularization of Medicine*, pp. 134–59.

Eminent Physician, *The Nurse's Guide: or, The Right Method of bringing up Young Children. To which is Added, an Essay on Preserving Health, and Prolonging Life* (London, 1729).

Falconer, W., *A Dissertation on the Influence of the Passions upon Disorders of the Body* (London, 1788).

The Female Aegis: or, The Duties of Women From Childhood to Old Age, and in Most Situations of Life Exemplified (London, 1798).

Fielding, H., *Tom Jones* (London, 1749).

Floyer, J., *Medicina gerocomica: or, The Galenic Art of Preserving Old Men's Healths* (London, 1724).

—, *The Ancient Psychrolousia Revived: or, An Essay to Prove Cold Bathing both Safe and Useful* (London, 1697).

—, *The Physician's Pulse Watch* (London 1707–19).

Foote, S., *A Treatise on the Passions, so far as they Regard the Stage* (London, 1747).

Fothergill, J., *Rules for the Preservation of Health* (London, 1762).

Garrick, D., *An Essay on Acting* (London, 1744).

Gaubius, H. D., *On the Passions: or A Philosophical Discourse Concerning the Duty and Office of Physicians in the Management and Cure of the Disorders of the Mind* (London, 1760).

Godwin, W., *An Enquiry Concerning Political Justice, and its Influence on General Virtue and Happiness* (Dublin, 1793).

Harris, J., *The Divine Physician: Prescribing Rules for the Prevention, and Cure of Most Diseases as well of the Body, as the Soul* (Norwich, 1709).

Harvey, W., M.D, 'The Anatomical Examination of the body of Thomas Parr', in R. Willis, *The Works of William Harvey* (London, 1847), pp. 589–92.

Hill, A., *The Works of the Late Aaron Hill* (London, 1754).

Hill, J., *The Actor: A Treatise on the Art of Playing* (London, 1750).

—, *The Old Man's Guide to Health and Longer Life* (London, 1764).

—, *The Virtues of Sage, in Lengthening Human Life: With Rules to Attain Old Age in Health and Cheerfulness* (London, 1765).

The Invalid: with the Obvious Means of Enjoying Health and Long Life (London, 1804).

Johnson, J., *The Economy of Health* (London, 1837).

Johnson, S., *A Dictionary of the English Language* (London, 1755).

Lloyd, R., *The Actor. A Poetical Epistle to Bonnell Thornton, Esq.* (London, 1760).

Locke, J., *Essay Concerning Human Understanding* (London, 1690).

Lucas, R., *An Enquiry after Happiness* (London, 1734).

Lynch, B., *A Guide to Health Through the Various Stages of Life* (London, 1744).

Massey, W. (trans.), *Tully's Compendious Treatise of Old Age* (London, 1753).

Maynwaringe, E., *The Method and Means of Enjoying Health, Vigour, and Long Life* (London, 1683).

The Miracle of Miracles, Being a Historical Account of the Birth, Parentage, Education and Long Long Life, of Dame Jane Scrimshaw (London, 1711).

Monro, J., *Remarks on Dr. Battie's Treatise on Madness* (London, 1758).

Nisbet, W., *The New Domestic Medicine* (London, 1809).

Partridge, J., *Defectio geniturarum, Being an Essay Toward the Reviving and Proving the True Old Principles of Astrology Hitherto Neglected or at Leastwise Not Observed or Understood* (London, 1697).

Pickering, R., *Reflections upon Theatrical Expression in Tragedy* (London, 1755).

Priestley, J., *Observations on Respiration, and the use of the Blood* (London, 1776).

Rush, B., 'An Account of the State of the Body and Mind in Old Age', in J. Sinclair, *The Code of Health and Longevity* (London, 1807), pp. 514–31.

Samber, R., *Long Livers: A Curious History of Such Persons of both Sexes who have Liv'd Several Ages, and Grown Young Again* (London, 1722).

Steele, R., *A Discourse Concerning Old-Age: Tending to the Instruction, Caution, and Comfort of Aged Persons* (London, 1688).

Sterne, L., 'On Chearfulness', in *The Works of Laurence Sterne* (Dublin, 1774), p. 54.

Stolberg, M., 'Female Menopause and Male Climacteric in Pre-modern Medicine', paper presented at *(Re)constructing the Aging Body: Western Medical Cultures and Gender 1600–2000*, Mainz, Germany, 26–8 September 2008.

Strother, E., *An Essay on Sickness and Health* (London, 1725).

—, *The Family Companion for Health* (London, 1729).

Swineburne, H., *A Treatise of Spousals, or Matrimonial Contracts* (London, 1711).

Temple, W., 'Of Health and Long Life', in *The Works of Sir William Temple* (London, 1710), vol. I, pt. 3, pp. 272–90.

The Best and Easiest Method of Preserving Uninterrupted Health to Extreme Old Age (London, 1748), pp. 189–90.

Thicknesse, P., *The Valetudinarians Bath Guide. Or, The Means of Obtaining Long Life and Health* (London, 1780).

'True Penitent', *The Folly, Sin, and Danger of Marrying Widows, and Old Women in General, Demonstrated and Earnestly address'd to the Batchelors of Great Britain* (London, 1746).

Trusler, Dr., *A Sure Way to Strengthen Life with Vigour: Particularly in Old Age; the Result of Experience* (London, 1819).

Tryon, T., *The Way to Health, Long Life and Happiness* (London, 1691).

—, *The Knowledge of a Man's Self, the Surest Guide to The True Worship of God, and Good Government of the Mind and Body* (London, 1704).

Ward, E., *The Amorous Bugbears: Or, the Humours of a Masquerade* (London, 1725).

Wesley, J., *Primitive Physick: or, an Easy and Natural Method of Curing Most Diseases* (London, 1747).

Wilson, E. (trans.), *Hufeland's Art of Prolonging Life* (London, 1853).

Woolley, H., *The Gentlewoman's Companion* (London, 1689).

Secondary Material

Abbott, M., *Life Cycles in England 1560–1720: Cradle to Grave* (London and New York: Routledge, 1996).

Agnew, J. C., *Worlds Apart: The Market and the Theatre in Anglo-American Thought, 1550–1750* (Cambridge: Cambridge University Press, 1986).

Arber, S., and J. Ginn (eds), *Connecting Gender & Ageing: A Sociological Approach* (Buckingham, Philadelphia, PA: Open University Press, 1995).

Armstrong, N., and L. Tennenhouse, *The Ideology of Conduct: Essays on Literature and the History of Sexuality* (New York and London: Routledge, 1987).

Atchley, R. C., *Social Forces and Aging: An Introduction to Social Gerontology* (Belmont, CA, 2000).

—, 'Continuity Theory, Self, and Social Structure', in C. D. Ryff and V. W. Marshall, *The Self and Society in Aging Processes* (New York: Springer Publishing Company, 1999), pp. 94–121.

Auf dem Keller, C., *Textual Structures in Eighteenth-Century Newspaper Advertising: A Corpus-Based Study of Medical Advertisements and Book Advertisements* (Aachen: Shaker Verlag GmbH, 2004).

Barker, H., *Newspapers, Politics, and Public Opinion in Late Eighteenth-Century England* (Oxford: Clarendon Press, 1998).

Barker-Benfield, G. J., *The Culture of Sensibility: Sex and Society in Eighteenth-Century Britain* (London and Chicago: University of Chicago Press, 1992).

Barrell, J., *The Birth of Pandora and the Division of Knowledge* (Basingstoke: Palgrave Macmillan, 1992).

Beam, A. C. L., 'Should I as Yet Call You Old?' Testing the Boundaries of Female Old Age in Early Modern England', in E. Campbell (ed.), *Growing Old in Early Modern Europe: Cultural Representations* (Aldershot and Burlington, VT: Ashgate Publishing Limited, 2006), pp. 98–114.

Ben-Amos, I. K., *Adolescence and Youth in Early Modern England* (New Haven, CT and London: Yale University Press, 1994).

Black, J., *The English Press in the Eighteenth Century* (London: Taylor & Francis, 1987).

Botelho, L. A., 'Images of Old Age in Early Modern Cheap Print: Women, Witches and the Poisonous Female Body', in L. A. Botelho, K. Kitteridge and S. Ottaway (eds), *Power and Poverty: Old Age in the Pre-Industrial Past* (London: Praeger, 2002), pp. 226–40.

—, 'Old age and menopause in rural women of early modern Suffolk', in L. Botelho and P. Thane (eds), *Women and Aging in British Society since 1500* (London: Pearson Education, 2001).

—, 'When the Healer becomes the Patient: Old Age and Illness in the Life of Elizabeth Freke, 1641–1714', in C. Streubel (ed.), *Aging Stories: Narrative Constructions of Age and Gender* (Frankfurt and New York, 2009).

Botelho, L., and P. Thane, *Women and Aging in British Society since 1500* (London: Pearson Education, 2001).

Bowling, A., S. See-Tai, E. Shah, G. Zahava and P. Solanki, 'Attributes of Age-Identity', *Ageing & Society*, 25 (2005), pp. 479–500.

Brewer, J., *The Pleasures of the Imagination: English Culture in the Eighteenth Century* (London: Farrar, Straus and Giroux, 1997).

Brosch, R., 'Spectacular Emotions: Edmund Burke's Redefintion of Visible Identity', in Gobel, Schabio and Windisch (eds), *Engendering Images of Man in the Long Eighteenth Century* (Trier: WVT Wissenschaftlicher Verlag, 2001), pp. 22–37.

Campbell, E. (ed.), *Growing Old in Early Modern Europe: Cultural Representations.* (Aldershot and Burlington, VT: Ashgate Publishing Limited, 2006).

Carter, P., 'Men about Town: Representations of Foppery and Masculinity in Early Eighteenth-Century Urban Society', in H. Barker and E. Chalus (eds), *Gender in Eighteenth-Century England: Roles, Representations and Responsibilities* (London and New York: Longman, 1997), pp. 31–57.

—, *Men and the Emergence of Polite Society, Britain 1660–1800* (London: Pearson Education, 2001).

Casler, J. M, 'Aging and Opportunity: Growing Older in Clara Reeve's *School for Widows* (1791)', *Journal of Aging and Identity*, 4:2 (June 1999), pp. 291–310.

Castle, T., *Masquerade and Civilization: the Carnivalesque in Eighteenth-Century English Culture and Fiction* (Stanford, CA: Stanford University Press, 1986).

Clark, S., 'Inversion, Misrule and the Meaning of Witchcraft', *Past and Present*, 87 (May 1980), pp. 98–127.

—, *Thinking with Demons: The Idea of Witchcraft in Early Modern Europe* (Oxford, 2003).

Cohen, M., '"Manners" Make the Man: Politeness, Chivalry, and the Construction of Masculinity, 1750–1830', *Journal of British Studies*, 44 (April 2005), pp. 312–29.

Connell, R. W., *Masculinities* (Cambridge: Cambridge University Press, 1995).

Cooke, W., *The Elements of Dramatic Criticism* (London: Printed for G. Kearsly, 1775).

—, *The Life and Death of David Garrick, Esq.* (London, 1779).

Cunningham, A., 'Boerhaave's Medical System, and Why it was Adopted in Edinburgh', in A. Cunningham and R. French (eds), *The Medical Enlightenment of the Eighteenth Century* (Cambridge: Cambridge University Press, 1990), pp. 40–66.

Daston, L., 'Historical Epistemology', in J. Chandler et al. (eds), *Questions of Evidence: Proof, Practice, and Persuasion Across the Disciplines* (Chicago, IL: University of Chicago Press Journals, 1994).

Davidoff, L., and C. Hall, *Family Fortunes: Men and Women of the English Middle Class, 1780–1850* (Chicago, IL: University of Chicago Press, 1987).

Davies, K. M., 'Continuity and Change in Literary Advice on Marriage', in R. B. Outhwaite (ed.), *Marriage and Society: Studies in the Social History of Marriage* (London: Europa, 1981), pp. 58–80.

Davies, T., *Memoirs of the Life of David Garrick* (London, 1780).

Dove, M., *The Perfect Age of Man's Life* (Cambridge: Cambridge University Press, 1986).

Downer, A., 'Nature to Advantage Dressed: Eighteenth-Century Acting', *Publications of the Modern Language Association of America*, 58 (December 1943), 4:1, pp. 1009–30.

Downie, J. A., and T. N. Corns (eds), *Telling People What to Think: Early Eighteenth-Century Periodicals from the Review to the Rambler* (London: Routledge, 1993).

Duden, B., 'Medicine and the History of the Body: The Lady of the Court', in J. Lachmund and G. Stollberg (eds), *The Social Construction of Illness: Illness and Medical Knowledge in Past and Present* (Stuttgart: Koch, Neff & Oetinger & Co, 1992), pp. 39–52.

'Eminent Physician', *The Nurse's Guide ... To which is Added, an Essay on Preserving Health, and Prolonging Life* (London, 1729).

Evans, J. G., 'Geriatric Medicine: A Brief History', *British Medical Journal*, 315 (1997), pp. 1075–77.

Feist, T., *The Stationer's Voice: The English Almanac Trade in the Early Eighteenth Century* (Philadelphia, PA: Amer Philosophical Society, 2005).

Figlio, K., 'The Historiography of Scientific Medicine: An Invitation to the Human Sciences', *Comparative Studies in Society and History*, 19:3 (July 1977), pp. 262–86.

Fischer-Lichte, E., 'Theatre and the Civilizing Process: An Approach to the History of Acting', in T. Postlethwait and B. A. McConachie (eds), *Interpreting the Theatrical Past: Essays in the Historiography of Performance* (Iowa: University of Iowa Press, 1989), pp. 23–45.

Fletcher, A., *Gender, Sex and Subordination in England 1500–1800* (New Haven, CT and London: Yale University Press, 1995).

Flynn, C. H., 'Defoe's Idea of Conduct: Ideological Fictions and Fictional Reality', in N. Armstrong and L. Tennenhouse (eds), *The Ideology of Conduct: Essays on Literature and the History of Sexuality* (New York and London: Routledge, 1987).

Foyster, E. A., *Manhood in Early Modern England: Honour, Sex and Marriage* (London and New York, 1999);

Freeman, L. A., *Character's Theater: Genre and Identity on the Eighteenth-Century English Stage* (Philadelphia, PA, 2002).

French, H., and M. Rothery, 'Upon your Entry into the World: Masculine Values and the Threshold of Adulthood among Landed Elites in England 1680–1800', *Social History*, 33:4 (November 2008), pp. 402–22.

Gallagher, C., and T. Laqueur (eds), *The Making of the Modern Body: Sexuality and Society in the Nineteenth Century* (Los Angeles, CA and London; University of California Press, 1987).

Gillis, J., *Youth and History: Tradition and Change in European age Relations, 1770–Present* (London: Academic Press, 1981).

Gilman, S. L., *Difference and Pathology: Stereotypes of Sexuality, Race, and Madness* (Ithaca, NY and London: Cornell University Press, 1985).

Goodden, A., *The Eighteenth Century Body: Art History, Literature, Medicine* (London: Peter Lang, 2002).

Goring, P., *The Rhetoric of Sensibility in Eighteenth-Century Culture* (Cambridge: Cambridge University Press, 2005).

Gowing, L., *Common Bodies: Women, Touch & Power in Seventeenth-Century England* (Oxford: Yale University Press, 2003).

Gregory, J., '*Homo Religious:* Masculinity and Religion in the Long Eighteenth Century', in T. Hitchcock and M. Cohen (eds), *English Masculinities 1660–1800* (London and New York: Longman, 1999), pp. 85–110.

Gruman, G. J., 'A History of Ideas about the Prolongation of Life: The Evolution of Prolongevity Hypotheses to 1800', *Transactions of the American Philosophical Society*, 54:9 (1966), pp. 6–85.

Guerrini, A., *Obesity and Depression in the Enlightenment: the Life and Times of George Cheyne* (London: University of Oklahoma Press, 1999).

Gullette, M. M., 'Male Midlife Sexuality in a Gerontocratic Economy: The Privileged Stage of the Long Midlife in Nineteenth-Century Age Ideology', *Journal of the History of Sexuality*, 5:1 (July 1994), pp. 58–89.

—, 'From Life Storytelling to Age Autobiography', *Journal of Aging Studies*, 18 (February 2003), pp. 101–11.

—, *Aged by Culture* (Chicago, IL: University of Chicago Press, 2004).

Hareven, T. K., 'The Life Course and Aging in Historical Perspective', in T. K. Hareven and K. J. Adams (eds), *Ageing and Life Course Transitions: An Interdisciplinary Perspective* (London and New York: Routledge, 1982), pp. 1–26.

K. Harvey, '"The Majesty of the Masculine-Form": Multiplicity and Male Bodies in Eighteenth Century Erotica', in T. Hitchcock and M. Cohen (eds), *English Masculinities* (London: Longman, 1999), pp. 193–214.

—, 'The Substance of Sexual Difference: Change and Persistence in Representations of the Body in c18 England', *Gender & History*, 14:2 (August 2002), pp. 202–23.

Haycock, D. B., *This Mortal Coil: A Short History of Living Longer* (New Haven, CT and London: Yale University Press, 2008).

Hiffernan, P., *Reflections on the Structure, and Passions of Man* (London, 1748).

—, *The Dramatic Genius* (London: printed for the author, 1770).

Hitchcock, T., *English Sexualities, 1700–1800* (Basingstoke and London: Palgrave Macmillan, 1997).

Hitchcock, T., and M. Cohen (eds), *English Masculinities 1660–1800* (London and New York: Longman, 1999).

Jacyna, S., 'Medicine in Transformation, 1800–1849', in W. F. Bynum, A. Hardy, S. Jacyna, C. Lawrence and E. M Tansey (eds), *The Western Medical Tradition 1800–2000* (Cambridge: Cambridge University Press, 2006), pp. 11–101.

Jones, C., and R. Porter (eds), *Reassessing Foucault: Power, Medicine and the Body* (London and New York: Routeledge, 1994).

Jordanova, L., *The Sense of a Past in Eighteenth-Century Medicine* (Reading: University of Reading, 1999).

Katz, S., 'A New Biopolitics of Age: Enhancement, Performance, Function', paper presented at *(Re)interpreting the Aging Body: Western Medical Cultures and Gender 1600–2000*, Mainz, Germany, 26–8 September 2008).

Kaufman, G., and G. Elder, 'Revisiting Age Identity: a research note', *Journal of Aging Studies*, 16:2 (May 2002), pp. 169–76.

Kertzner, D., and J. Keith (eds), *Age and Anthropological Theory* (Ithaca, NY and London: Cornell University Press, 1984).

Kitteridge, K., 'The Ag'd Dame to Venery Inclin'd: Images of Sexual Older Women in Eighteenth-Century Britain', in L. A. Botelho, K. Kitteridge and S. Ottaway (eds), *Power and Poverty: Old Age in the Pre-Industrial Past* (London: Praeger, 2002), pp. 248–59.

Klein, L. E., 'Politeness and the Interpretation of the British Eighteenth Century'. Historiographical Review, *Historical Journal*, 45:4 (2002), pp. 869–98.

—, *Shaftesbury and the Culture of Politeness: Moral Discourse and Cultural Politics in Early Eighteenth-Century England* (Cambridge: Cambridge University Press, 1994), p. 4.

Kohli, M., 'The World We Forgot: A Historical Review of the Life Course', in V. W. Marshall (ed.), *Later Life: The Social Psychology of Aging* (Beverly Hills, London and New Delhi: Sage, 1986), pp. 271–303.

Kugler, A., '"I Feel Myself Decay Apace": Old Age in the Diary of Lady Sarah Cowper (1644–1720)', in L. Botelho and P. Thane (eds), *Women and Aging in British Society since 1500* (London: Pearson Education, 2001).

Laqueur, T., *Making Sex: The Body and Gender from the Greeks to Freud* (Cambridge, MA, and London: Harvard University Press, 1990).

Langford, P., *A Polite and Commercial People, England 1727–1780* (Oxford: Oxford University Press, 1989).

Laslett, P., *Family Life and Illicit Love in Earlier Generations: Essays in Historical Sociology* (Cambridge: Cambridge University Press, 1977).

—, 'The Significance of the Past in the Study of Ageing; Introduction to the Special Issue on History and Ageing', *Ageing and Society*, 4:4 (1984), pp. 379–89.

—, *A Fresh Map of Life: The Emergence of the Third Age* (London: Weidenfeld and Nicolson, 1989).

Lynch, D. S., *The Economy of Character: Novels, Market Culture, and the Business of Inner Meaning* (Chicago, IL and London: University of Chicago Press, 1998).

Markley, R., 'Sentimentality as Performance: Shaftesbury, Sterne, and the Theatrics of Virtue', in F. Nussbaum and L. Brown (eds), *The New Eighteenth Century* (New York and London: Routledge, 1987), pp. 210–30.

Marshall, B., 'Science, Medicine and Virility Surveillance: The New Biology of "Sexy Seniors"', paper presented at *(Re)constructing the Aging Body: Western Medical Cultures and Gender 1600–2000*, Mainz, Germany, 26–8 September2008.)

Marshall, D., 'Adam Smith and the Theatricality of Moral Sentiments', *Critical Inquiry*, 10:4 (June 1984), pp. 592–613.

—, *The Figure of Theater: Shaftesbury, Defoe, Adam Smith and George Eliot* (New York: Columbia University Press, 1986).

Martin, R., and J. Barresi, *Naturalization of the Soul: Self and Personal Identity in the Eighteenth Century* (London, 2000).

Mauss, M. (trans. W. D. Halls), 'A Category of the Human Mind: The Notion of the Person; the Notion of Self', in M. Carrithers, S. Collins and S. Lukes (eds), *The Category of the Person: Anthropology, Philosophy, History* (Cambridge: Cambridge University Press, 1985), pp. 1–25.

McCormack, M., *The Independent Man: Citizenship and Gender Politics in Georgian England* (Manchester: Manchester University Press, 2005).

McKenzie, A. T., 'The Countenance You Show Me: Reading the Passions in the Eighteenth Century', *Georgia Review*, 32:4 (Winter 1978), pp. 758–73.

Mullan, J., *Sentiment and Sociability: The Language of Feeling in the Eighteenth Century* (Oxford: Clarendon Press, 1988).

Munson Deats, S., and L. Tallen Lenker (eds), *Aging and Identity: A Humanities Perspective* (London: Greenwood Publishing Group, 1999).

Nussbaum, F., *The Autobiographical Subject: Gender and Ideology in Eighteenth-Century England* (Baltimore, MD and London, 1989).

Okin, S. M., 'Women and the Making of the Sentimental Family', *Philosophy and Public Affairs*, 11:1 (Winter 1982), pp. 65–88.

Ottaway, S., *The Decline of Life: Old Age in Eighteenth-Century England* (Cambridge: Cambridge University Press, 2004).

Otto, P., 'Performing the Resurrection: James Graham and the Multiplication of the Real', *Cultural and Social History*, 3:3 (2006), pp. 325–40.

Outhwaite, R. B., 'Problems and Perspectives in the History of Marriage', in R. B. Outhwaite, *Marriage and Society: Studies in the Social History of Marriage* (London: Europa, 1981), pp. 1–17.

Paulson, R., 'Life as Journey and as Theater: Two Eighteenth-Century Narrative Structures', *New Literary History*, 8:11 (Autumn 1976), pp. 43–58.

Pilloud, S., and M. Louis-Courvoisier, 'The Intimate Experience of the Body in the Eighteenth Century: Between Interiority and Exteriority', *Medical History*, 47 (October 2003), pp. 451–72.

Pittard, J., *Observations on Mr. Garrick's Acting* (London, 1758).

Poole, R., 'Give us our Eleven Days!' Calendar Reform in Eighteenth Century England', *Past and Present*, 149 (1995), pp. 95–139.

Porter, R., 'Lay Medical Knowledge in the Eighteenth-Century: The Evidence of the *Gentleman's Magazine*', *Medical History*, 29:2 (1985), pp. 138–68.

—, 'Civilization and Disease: Medical Ideology in the Enlightenment', in J. Black and J. Gregory (eds), *Culture, Politics and Society in Britain 1660–1800* (Manchester: Manchester University Press, 1991), pp. 154–83.

—, 'The Eighteenth Century', in L. I. Conrad, M. Neve, V. Nutton, R. Porter and A. Wear (eds), *The Western Medical Tradition 800 BC to AD 1800* (Cambridge: Cambridge University Press, 1995), pp. 371–477.

—, *Rewriting the Self: Histories from the Renaissance to the Present* (London: Psychology Press, 1997).

—, *Bodies Politic: Disease, Death and Doctors in Britain, 1650–1900* (Ithaca, NY: Cornell University Press, 2001).

—, *Flesh in the Age of Reason: How the Enlightenment Transformed the Way We See Our Bodies and Souls* (London: W. W. Norton & Co., 2003).

Ralley, R., 'Climacterical Years: Astrology and Ageing in Early Modern England', paper presented at the Early Modern Philosophy and the Scientific Imagination seminar, London, 19 June 2009.

Reddy, W. M., *The Navigation of Feeling: A Framework for the History of Emotions* (Cambridge: Cambridge University Press, 2001).

Rieder, P., 'Patients and Words: A Lay Medical Culture?', in G. S. Rousseau, M. Gill, D. Haycock and M. Herwig (eds), *Framing and Imagining Disease in Cultural History* (Basingstoke: Palgrave Macmillan, 2003), pp. 215–26.

Riley, M. W. (ed.), *Aging from Birth to Death: Interdisciplinary Perspectives* (Boudler: Westview Press, 1979).

Roach, J. R., *The Player's Passion: Studies in the Science of Acting* (Newark, London and Toronto: University of Delaware Press, 1985).

Roberts, M. M., 'A Physic against Death: Eternal Life and the Enlightenment – Gender and Gerontology', in M. M. Roberts and R. Porter (eds), *Literature and Medicine During the Eighteenth Century* (London: Routledge, 1993), pp. 151–67.

Roebuck, J., 'When Does Old Age Begin? The Evolution of the English Definition', *Journal of Social History*, 12:3 (Spring 1979), pp. 416–29.

Rousseau, G. S., 'Nerves, Spirits, and Fibres: Towards Defining the Origins of Sensibility', in R. F. Brissenden and J. C. Eade (eds), *Studies in the Eighteenth Century III* (Toronto and Buffalo: University of Toronto Press, 1976), pp. 137–58.

—, 'J. S. Hill, Universal Genius *Manqué*: Remarks on his Life and Times, with a Checklist of his Works', in J. A. L. Lemay and G. S. Rousseau (eds), *The Renaissance Man in the Eighteenth Century* (Los Angeles, CA, 1978), pp. 45–129.

—, 'Science books and their readers in the eighteenth century', in I. Rivers (ed.), *Books and their Readers in Eighteenth-Century England* (Leicester, 1982), pp. 197–237.

— (ed.), *The Languages of Psyche: Mind and Body in Enlightenment Thought* (Berkeley and Los Angeles, CA and London, 1990).

Ryff, C. D., and V. W. Marshall (eds), *The Self and Society in Aging Processes* (New York: Springer Publishing Company, 1999).

Schafer, D., *Old Age and Disease in Early Modern Medicine* (London: Pickering & Chatto, 2011).

Shepard, A., *Meanings of Manhood in Early Modern England* (Oxford: Oxford University Press, 2003).

—, 'From Anxious Patriarchs to Refined Gentlemen? Manhood in Britain, circa 1500–1700', *Journal of British Studies*, 44 (April 2005), pp. 281–95.

Shevelow, K., *Women and Print Culture: The Construction of Femininity in the Early Periodical* (London and New York: Taylor & Francis, 1989).

Shoemaker, R. B., *Gender in English Society, 1650–1850: The Emergence of Separate Spheres?* (London: Longman, 1998).

Shuttleton, D. E., '"Pamela's Library": Samuel Richardson and Dr. Cheyne's "Universal Cure"', *Eighteenth-Century Life*, 23:1 (1999), pp. 59–79.

Smith, R., *Fontana History of the Human Sciences* (London: Fontana Press, 1997), Part III: 'The Long Eighteenth Century'.

Stallybrass, P., and A. White, *The Politics and Poetics of Transgression* (London: Taylor & Francis, 1986).

Stepan, N. L., 'Race, Gender, Science and Citizenship', *Gender and History*, 10 (1998).

Tadmor, N., 'The Concept of the Household-Family in Eighteenth-Century England', *Past and Present*, 151 (May 1996), pp. 111–40.

Taylor, C., *Sources of the Self: The Making of Modern Identity* (Cambridge, 1989).

—, 'The Person', in M. Carrithers, S. Collins and S. Lukes (eds), *The Category of the Person: Anthropology, Philosophy, History* (Cambridge: Cambridge University Press, 1995), pp. 257–81.

Taylor, J., *Annals of Health and Long Life* (London, 1818).

Taylor, J., 'The Old, Old, Very Old Man: or The Age and Long Life of Thomas Parr', in *Caulfield's Edition of Curious Tracts* (London, 1635; London, 1794).

Thane, P., *Old Age in English History: Past Experiences, Present Issues* (Oxford: Oxford University Press, 2000).

Thomas, K., 'Age and Authority in Early Modern England', *Proceedings of the British Academy*, 62 (1976), pp. 205–48.

Tosh, J., 'Masculinities in an Industrialising Society: Britain 1800–1914', *Journal of British Studies*, 44 (April 2005), pp. 330–42.

Troyansky, D. G, 'Historical Research into Ageing, Old Age and Older People', in A. Jamieson, S. Harper and C. Victor (eds), *Critical Approaches to Ageing and Later Life* (Philadelphia, PA: Open University Press, 1997), pp. 49–62.

Wahrman, D., *The Making of the Modern Self: Identity and Culture in Eighteenth-Century England* (New Haven, CT and London: Yale University Press, 2004).

Walters, A. N., 'Conversation Pieces: Science and Politeness in Eighteenth-century England', *History of Science*, 35:2:108 (June 1997), pp. 121–54.

Warner, R. (ed.), *Original Letters* (Bath and London, 1817).

Watt, I., *The Rise of the Novel* (Berkeley, CA: University of California Press, 1957).

Wear, A., 'Medicine in Early Modern Europe, 1500–1700', in L. I. Conrad, M. Neve, V. Nutton, R. Porter and A. Wear (eds), *The Western Medical Tradition 800 BC to AD 1800* (Cambridge: Cambridge University Press, 1995), pp. 215–370.

Wilson, A., 'The Politics of Medical Improvement in Early Hanoverian London', in A. Cunningham and R. French (eds), *The Medical Enlightenment of the Eighteenth Century* (Cambridge: Cambridge University Press, 1990), pp. 4–39.

Woods, L., *Garrick Claims the Stage: Acting as Social Emblem in Eighteenth-Century England* (Westport, CT and London: Greenwood Press, 1984).

INDEX